GYNECOLOGIC ULTRASOUND
A Problem-Based Approach

GYNECOLOGIC ULTRASOUND
A Problem-Based Approach

Beryl R. Benacerraf, MD

*Clinical Professor of Radiology and Obstetrics and Gynecology and
  Reproductive Biology*
Harvard Medical School
Radiologist
Brigham and Women's Hospital
Consultant in OB-GYN
Brigham and Women's Hospital and Massachusetts General Hospital
Boston, Massachusetts

Steven R. Goldstein, MD

Professor of Obstetrics and Gynecology
New York University School of Medicine
Director, Gynecologic Ultrasound
Co-Director, Bone Densitometry
New York University Langone Medical Center
New York, New York

Yvette S. Groszmann, MD, MPH

Clinical Instructor in Obstetrics, Gynecology, and Reproductive Biology
Harvard Medical School, Brigham and Women's Hospital
Boston, Massachusetts

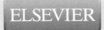

ELSEVIER
SAUNDERS

1600 John F. Kennedy Blvd.
Ste 1800
Philadelphia, PA 19103-2899

GYNECOLOGIC ULTRASOUND: A PROBLEM-BASED APPROACH   ISBN: 978-1-4377-3794-3
Copyright © 2014 by Saunders, an imprint of Elsevier Inc.

Notices

Knowledge and best practice in this field are constantly changing. As new research and experience broaden our understanding, changes in research methods, professional practices, or medical treatment may become necessary.

Practitioners and researchers must always rely on their own experience and knowledge in evaluating and using any information, methods, compounds, or experiments described herein. In using such information or methods they should be mindful of their own safety and the safety of others, including parties for whom they have a professional responsibility.

With respect to any drug or pharmaceutical products identified, readers are advised to check the most current information provided (i) on procedures featured or (ii) by the manufacturer of each product to be administered, to verify the recommended dose or formula, the method and duration of administration, and contraindications. It is the responsibility of practitioners, relying on their own experience and knowledge of their patients, to make diagnoses, to determine dosages and the best treatment for each individual patient, and to take all appropriate safety precautions.

To the fullest extent of the law, neither the Publisher nor the authors, contributors, or editors assume any liability for any injury and/or damage to persons or property as a matter of products liability, negligence or otherwise, or from any use or operation of any methods, products, instructions, or ideas contained in the material herein.

Library of Congress Cataloging-in-Publication Data

Benacerraf, Beryl R., author.
Gynecologic ultrasound: a problem-based approach / Beryl R. Benacerraf, Steven R. Goldstein, Yvette S. Groszmann.
     p. ; cm.
   Includes bibliographical references and index.
   ISBN 978-1-4377-3794-3 (hardcover : alk. paper)
   I. Goldstein, Steven R., author. II. Groszmann, Yvette S., author. III. Title.
   [DNLM: 1. Genital Diseases, Female--ultrasonography. 2. Ultrasonography--methods. WP 141]
   RG107.5.U4
   618.1'07543--dc23   2013046132

Executive Content Strategist: Helene Caprari
Content Development Specialist: Joanie Milnes
Publishing Services Manager: Jeff Patterson
Project Manager: Clay S. Broeker
Design Direction: Louis Forgione

Printed in China

Last digit is the print number: 9 8 7 6 5 4 3 2 1

Working together
to grow libraries in
developing countries

www.elsevier.com • www.bookaid.org

This book is dedicated to my husband, Peter Libby, who gave me love, encouragement, inspiration, and support throughout my life; and to my children, Oliver and Brigitte Libby, who make me proud and complete my life.
Beryl Benacerraf

This book is dedicated to the late Robert F. Porges, MD, who believed in me when some others didn't and gave me the opportunity to prove I "could," and it is dedicated as well to the very-much-alive Wendy J. Sarasohn, who has connected to the part of me now able to see the "rainbows."
Steven Goldstein

I would like to dedicate this to my parents, Dr. Roberto Groszmann and Aida Groszmann, for giving me a wonderful life. Additionally, I would like to thank David Sella, my lifelong friend and talented photographer. Lastly, I need to thank Dr. Beryl Benacerraf. She is a brilliant physician and a wonderful colleague, and I am lucky to call her my mentor.
Yvette Groszmann

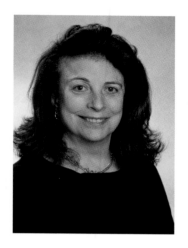

Beryl R. Benacerraf

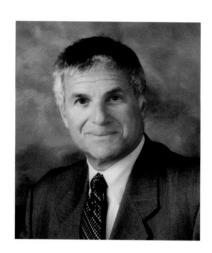

Steven R. Goldstein

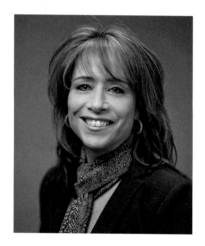

Yvette S. Groszmann

Receiving her MD in 1976 from Harvard Medical School, **Beryl R. Benacerraf** went on to complete her internship at Peter Bent Brigham Hospital, her residency at Massachusetts General Hospital, and her fellowship in ultrasound and computed tomography at Brigham and Women's Hospital. During her 34-year academic affiliation with Harvard Medical School, she has risen to the rank of clinical professor in obstetrics, gynecology, and reproductive biology and radiology. From 1991 through 1993, Dr. Benacerraf was co-director of high-risk obstetric ultrasound at Brigham and Women's Hospital, and from 1993 through 1999 she was director of the obstetric ultrasound unit at Massachusetts General Hospital.

Active in the ultrasound community, Dr. Benacerraf has directed and organized a host of postgraduate ultrasound courses. Among her many roles in the ultrasound community, she is an elected fellow of the American College of Radiology and the Society of Radiologists in Ultrasound, was treasurer of the World Federation for Ultrasound in Medicine and Biology for 7 years, is the current president-elect of the American Institute of Ultrasound in Medicine, and is a board member of the International Society of Ultrasound in Obstetrics and Gynecology. Dr. Benacerraf is also the medical director and president of Diagnostic Ultrasound Associates, PC, a medical practice that she founded in 1982. She served as Editor in Chief of the *Journal of Ultrasound in Medicine* from 2000 to 2010. Her contributions to the field of diagnostic ultrasound have been recognized by the Ian Donald Gold Medal of the International Society of Ultrasound in Obstetrics and Gynecology, the Frye Award, and the Holmes award (both from the American Institute of Ultrasound). She was selected to deliver the Silver Lecture at Barnard College in 2007, and she received the 2008 Marie Curie Award from the Association of Women Radiologists. In 2010, she was the recipient of the Larry Mack award for lifetime achievement in ultrasound research from the Society of Radiologists in Ultrasound.

Having authored more than 260 peer-reviewed articles, she has focused her research on the detection and significance of fetal anomalies. Dr. Benacerraf did the original research that linked nuchal thickening directly to an increased risk for fetal Down syndrome and developed the genetic sonogram, both of which have changed the way all pregnant women are currently screened for fetal Down syndrome. She has also made important contributions to the implementation of 3-D ultrasound in both obstetrics and gynecology. She has contributed chapters to many textbooks in the field and is the sole author of *Ultrasound of Fetal Syndromes*, recently published in its second edition. More recently, she has taken a special interest in ultrasound of gynecologic patients, in particular those with chronic pelvic pain.

Steven R. Goldstein, MD, is a Magna Cum Laude graduate of Colgate University with a Baccalaureate degree in Biology. He graduated from the New York University School of Medicine and did an internship in Obstetrics and Gynecology at Parkland Memorial Hospital in Dallas, Texas. He did a residency in Obstetrics and Gynecology at New York University Affiliated Hospitals/ Bellevue Hospital Center. Thereafter he joined the faculty of the Department of Obstetrics and Gynecology at New York University School of Medicine, rising to his current rank of Professor of Obstetrics and Gynecology, a tenured full-time academic position. However, in this capacity, he maintains a half-time private practice as a generalist in Obstetrics and Gynecology in the Faculty Practice suites at New York University.

His longstanding interests in OB-GYN ultrasound have led him to his current position as Director of Gynecologic Ultrasound at New York University Medical Center. He is a Fellow of the American Institute of Ultrasound in Medicine and is currently President of this national organization. He is a past President of the North American Menopause Society. He served on the Board of Directors of the American Registry of Diagnostic Medical Sonographers, having prepared the test and administered policy for the certification of over 40,000 sonographers nationwide. He is a past Chairman of the American College of Obstetrics and Gynecology, New York section. He was author of their Technical Bulletin *Ultrasound in Gynecology* as well as the author of their practice guidelines on SERMs (selective estrogen receptor modulators). He serves as the liaison physician from the American College of Obstetrics and Gynecology to the Women's Health Imaging Panel of the American College of Radiology. He has been an examiner for the American Board of Obstetrics and Gynecology.

His pioneering work in menopausal and perimenopausal ultrasound led him into design of uterine safety studies for several Selective Estrogen Receptor Modulators. In addition he is the Co-Director of the Bone Densitometry Unit at NYU Langone Medical Center. Clinically, his practice has evolved into issues of menopausal and perimenopausal medicine with particular interest in ultrasound applications for both adnexal masses and abnormal bleeding.

He has authored textbooks titled *Endovaginal Ultrasound* and *Ultrasound in Gynecology*. More recently, he authored *Imaging in the Infertile Couple* and *Textbook of Perimenopausal Gynecology*. He is one of the most highly recognized and regarded individuals in the field of vaginal probe ultrasound worldwide. He has authored more than 60 chapters in textbooks and more than 80 original research articles. He has been a guest faculty member, invited speaker, visiting professor, or course director more than 400 times throughout the United States and the world.

Dr. Goldstein has a long history as an adviser and consultant to the pharmaceutical industry. He has been on gynecologic advisory boards and/or consulted for Amgen, Bayer, Boehringer Ingelheim, Eli Lilly, Merck, GlaxoSmithKline, Novo Nordisk, Wyeth, Procter & Gamble, Warner Chilcott, Shionogi, QuatRx, Depomed, and Pfizer. He has represented Eli Lilly, Pfizer, and Mirabilis Medica in their appearances before FDA Advisory Boards. He has designed studies of uterine safety for Eli Lilly, Wyeth, Pfizer, and GlaxoSmithKline. He holds two patents in the medical device arena. He was director of a publicly traded ultrasound company, SonoSite, Inc., from its inception until its sale to Fuji Medical in 2012.

He resides in New York City.

Yvette S. Groszmann attended Tufts University and graduated with a BS in Biopsychology. She obtained her medical degree in 2000 from the University of Connecticut, as well as a Master's in Public Health. She then completed a residency in Obstetrics and Gynecology at Pennsylvania Hospital in Philadelphia. Her residency training emphasized the importance of ultrasound as part of the routine practice of obstetrics and gynecology. As a result, she received considerable training and practice in ultrasound during her time at Pennsylvania Hospital. After completing her formal training, she joined a multispecialty medical group in Boston as a full-time obstetrician-gynecologist with hospital appointments at Brigham and Women's Hospital and Faulkner Hospital. In 2009, Dr. Groszmann left her practice as a generalist to do a fellowship in diagnostic ultrasound under the guidance of Dr. Beryl Benacerraf. She joined Diagnostic Ultrasound Associates in 2010 and continues her affiliation with Brigham and Women's Hospital. Dr. Groszmann enjoys teaching, and she received a teaching award during residency. She is currently a clinical instructor at Harvard Medical School and teaches gynecologic ultrasound to the OB-GYN residents.

Dr. Groszmann is a fellow of the American College of Obstetrics and Gynecology and a member of the American Institute of Ultrasound in Medicine. She is board certified in Obstetrics and Gynecology.

Preface

This book is designed for the clinician as a practical approach to problem-solving for gynecologic patients. The book provides a stepwise and convenient guide to the diagnosis of gynecologic abnormalities for practitioners providing gynecologic care.

The book is organized by a listing of symptoms or findings that a practitioner might encounter when evaluating a patient sonographically (in the Contents section called *List of Differential Diagnoses*). These categories include a variety of topics, including pelvic pain, pelvic masses, and postmenopausal bleeding. Under each category, there is a list of differential diagnostic possibilities. For example, within pelvic pain, the differential diagnoses include appendicitis, ectopic pregnancy, hemorrhagic cyst, degenerating fibroid, and so on. The reader can select or refer to the specific disease or entity to go into a "mini-chapter" (there are 54 of these) and read more about that particular entity and its sonographic appearance, as well as review images illustrating it.

The 54 mini-chapters focus on each entity or diagnosis (such as hemorrhagic cyst, fibroid, or polyps) and contain abundant images (more than 600) from several patients to give comprehensive examples of the sonographic and Doppler findings for each of these findings or disease states. Each mini-chapter is arranged in a standard format that includes Synonyms/Description, Etiology, Ultrasound Findings, Differential Diagnosis, Clinical Aspects and Recommendations, and Suggested Reading. There is also a chapter on the normal ultrasound examination of the female pelvis, followed by a series of 26 test cases of abnormalities for readers to see what they have learned.

This book is not a standard textbook on gynecologic ultrasound, of which there are many excellent offerings. Most of these textbooks are constructed with separate chapters for each organ (such as the uterus, ovary, and fallopian tubes). Rather, this book is intended as a reference focused on problem solving. A clinician can consult the book to look up a specific symptom or finding and help narrow down the differential diagnoses to one correct entity.

This book is intended for radiologists, obstetricians/gynecologists, infertility specialists, emergency physicians, sonographers, and residents in OB-GYN and radiology who perform pelvic ultrasound. The book may also be useful to primary care physicians, nurse practitioners, physician's assistants, and other personnel who see patients with pelvic symptoms and order the imaging. The diagnoses are presented by symptom, differential diagnosis, and alphabetically for easy searching.

It is hoped that this book will give practitioners who take care of women with pelvic complaints a practical reference that will be useful in solving their diagnostic dilemmas.

Contents

Section 1 ENTITIES

A

Adenomyosis 3
Adhesions (Peritoneal Inclusion Cyst) 8
Appendiceal Mucocele 11
Atrophic Endometrium 14

B

Bladder Masses 15
Borderline Ovarian Tumor 21
Bowel Diseases 26
Brenner Tumor 32

C

Cervical Masses 34
Cesarean Scar Defect 39
Corpus Luteum and Hemorrhagic Cyst 43
Cyst, Clear 48
Cystadenofibroma 51

D

Dermoid Cyst 53
Dysgerminoma 56

E

Ectopic Pregnancy 58
Endometrial Carcinoma 65
Endometrial Hyperplasia and the Differential
    Diagnosis for Thick Endometrium 71
Endometriosis 76
Epidermoid Cyst 83

F

Fibroids 85
Fibroma (Ovarian), Thecoma, and Fibrothecoma 93

G

Granulosa Cell Tumor 96

H

Hematometra and Hematocolpos 98
Hydrosalpinx 104

I

Intrauterine Device Location, Abnormal 109
Intravenous Leiomyomatosis 114

L

Lymph Nodes, Enlarged 116

M

Metastatic Tumor to the Ovary 118
Mucinous Cystadenoma 122
Müllerian Duct Anomalies 125

O

Ovarian Calcifications 136
Ovarian Cancer (Epithelial) 137
Ovarian/Tubal Torsion 147
Ovarian Vein Thrombosis 153

P

Paratubal or Paraovarian Cysts 155
Pelvic Congestion Syndrome 157
Pelvic Kidney 159
Polycystic Ovaries 161
Polyps, Endometrial 163
Premature Ovarian Failure 170

R

Retained Products of Conception 172

S

Scarred Uterus and Asherman's Syndrome 177
Schwannoma 182
Serous Cystadenoma 184
Struma Ovarii 186

T

T-Shaped Uterus 189
Tarlov Cysts 192
Theca Lutein Cyst 194
Tube Carcinoma, Primary Fallopian 196
Tubo-Ovarian Abcess and Pelvic Inflammatory
    Disease 199

U

Ureteral Stone 203
Uterine Sarcoma 205

V

Vaginal Masses 209

Section 2 NORMAL PELVIC ULTRASOUND AND COMMON NORMAL VARIANTS

Normal Pelvic Ultrasound and Common
    Normal Variants 221

Section 3 CASE STUDIES FOR REVIEW

List of Differential Diagnoses

Pelvic Pain

Acute

Appendicitis or mucocele   11
Degenerating fibroid   85
Ectopic pregnancy   58
Hemorrhagic cyst   43
Ovarian/adnexal torsion   147
Ovarian torsion   147
Ovarian vein thrombosis   153
Tubo-ovarian abscess/PID   199
Ureteral stone   203

Chronic

Adenomyosis   3
Adhesions—peritoneal inclusion cyst—loculated fluid   8
Cystitis   15
Deep penetrating endometriosis   76
Endometriosis/endometrioma   76
Fibroids   85
Hydrosalpinx   104
Inflammatory bowel disease   26
IUD (abnormal location)   111
Pelvic congestion   157
Pseudomyxoma peritonei   11
Salpingitis   199

Pelvic Mass

Uterine

Adenomyosis   3
Degenerating fibroid   85
Fibroid   85
Hematometra/hematocolpos   98
Nabothian cyst   38
Sarcoma   205

Vaginal mass
   Fibroid   85 and 209
   Gartner's duct cyst   209
   Lymphoma   116 and 209
   Sarcoma   209
Cervical mass
   Cervical cancer   38
   Cervical fibroid   38 and 85
   Cervical lymphoma   38 and 116
   Cervical polyp   38 and 163
Complex cystic mass
   Appendiceal mucocele   11
   Corpus luteum   43
   Cystadenofibroma   51
   Decidualized endometrioma in pregnancy   76
   Ectopic pregnancy   58
   Endometrioma   76
   Epidermoid cyst   83
   Hemorrhagic cyst   43
   Hydrosalpinx   104
   Mucinous cystadenoma   122
   Ovarian malignancy (borderline or invasive)   137
   Serous cystadenoma   184
   Theca luteum cyst   194
   Tubal malignancy   196
   Tubo-ovarian abscess   199
Solid mass
   Appendiceal mucocele   11
   Bowel-related masses   26
   Brenner tumor   32
   Dermoid   53
   Dysgerminoma   56
   Endometriosis implants   76
   Enlarged lymph node (lymphoma)   116
   Epidermoid cyst   83
   Fibroma   93
   Granulosa cell tumor   96
   Hemorrhagic cyst (acute)   43
   Intravascular leiomyomatosis   109
   Massive ovarian edema   147
   Metastatic carcinoma   118
   Ovarian calcifications   136
   Ovarian malignancy (borderline or invasive)   137

Pelvic kidney   159
Schwannoma   182
Tarlov cysts (bilateral)   192
Theca cell tumor   194
Tubal malignancy   196

Clear cyst
Cystadenoma   122 and 184
Follicle/unilocular physiologic cyst   48
Paraovarian cyst   155

Adnexal mass with normal ovary documented
Appendiceal mucocele   11
Appendix- or bowel-related mass   11 and 26
Broad ligament fibroid   85
Ectopic pregnancy   58
Hydrosalpinx   104
Intravascular leiomyomatosis   109
Paratubal cyst   155
Pelvic kidney   159
Peritoneal inclusion cyst   8
Tubal malignancy   196
Tubo-ovarian abscess   199

Abnormal Bleeding

Premenopausal
Adenomyosis   3
C-section scar defect (with collected blood)   34
Endometrial carcinoma   65
Endometrial hyperplasia   71
Functional ovarian cyst   48
Hematuria—bladder masses   15
IUD (abnormal location)   111
Polyps   163
Retained products of conception   172

Postmenopausal bleeding
Atrophic endometrium   14
Endometrial carcinoma   65
Endometrial hyperplasia   71
Hematuria—bladder masses   15
"One more cycle"   221
Polyps   163

Amenorrhea
Asherman's syndrome   177
Excessive exercise/anorexia   No page reference

PCOS   161
Perimenopause   No page reference
Pregnancy   No page reference

Infertility

Asherman's syndrome   177
Hydrosalpinx or salpingitis   104 and 199
Lack of follicular development   170
Lack of normal maturation of the endometrium during the cycle   No page reference
Müllerian duct abnormalities   125
PCOS   161
Pelvic inflammatory disease   199
Premature ovarian failure   170
Submucous fibroid   85
T-shaped uterus   189
Tubal occlusion   No page reference
Uterine synechiae   177

Recurrent Pregnancy Loss—Possible Ultrasound Findings

Asherman's syndrome   177
Müllerian duct abnormalities—septate or subseptate, unicornuate, bicornuate
T-shaped uterus   125 and 189

Video Contents

Appendiceal Mucocele Video 1
Appendiceal Mucocele Video 2
Appendiceal Mucocele Video 3

Bowel-Related Masses Video 1

Endometrial Carcinoma Video 1

Endometriosis/Endometrioma Video 1
Endometriosis/Endometrioma Video 2

Endometriosis/Endometrioma Video 3
Endometriosis/Endometrioma Video 4
Endometriosis/Endometrioma Video 5

Ovarian Cancer (Epithelial) Video 1

Ovarian/Tubal Torsion, Edema (Massive) Video 1

Retained Products of Conception Video 1
Retained Products of Conception Video 2

Entities

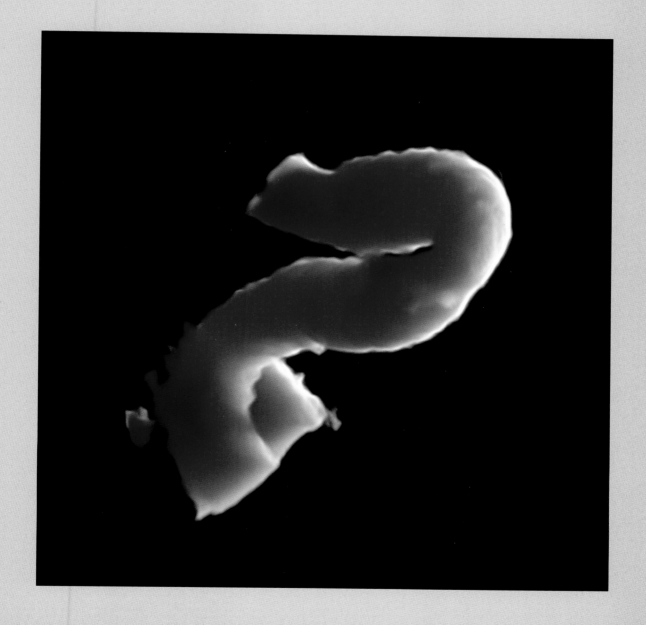

Adenomyosis

Synonyms/Description
Endometriosis of the uterus or myometrium

Etiology
Adenomyosis is defined pathologically when endometrial glands and stroma are found in the myometrium, distant from the endometrial cavity itself. This ectopic endometrial tissue has the ability to induce hypertrophy of the surrounding myometrium. This process can be focal or diffuse and thus accounts for the variability in the ultrasound appearances noted. The endometrium-myometrium junctional zone is jagged and fuzzy because the endometrial mucosa essentially invades the underlying myometrium, thus blurring the interface between these two, typically distinct zones. (This may be focal or global.)

Ultrasound Findings
Generalized Adenomyosis
The uterus is typically enlarged and globular with heterogeneous myometrium, which is typically wider on one side than the other. The heterogeneous myometrium often contains myometrial cysts, which likely represent areas of glandular dilatation or hemorrhage caused by repeated bleeding. These cysts are also frequently seen in a subendometrial location.

Adenomyoma
An adenomyoma appears as a focal, somewhat circumscribed island of heterogeneity in the myometrium, suggesting a fibroid, but typically without clear borders. When the borders are sharp, one cannot distinguish an adenomyoma from a fibroid. The adenomyoma may project into the cavity in the form of a broad-based polyp (polypoid adenomyoma).

Three-dimensional (3-D) ultrasound is helpful to demonstrate the multitude of linear hyperechoic bands emanating from the endometrium into the myometrium, producing the shaggy outline of the endometrial cavity on 3-D coronal view of the uterus.

Although magnetic resonance imaging (MRI) has been useful for diagnosing adenomyosis, it is unnecessary because ultrasound has similar accuracy. A comparison between ultrasound and MRI was reported using 23 articles (involving 2312 women). Transvaginal ultrasound had a sensitivity and specificity of 72% and 81%, respectively, whereas MRI had a sensitivity and specificity of 77% and 89%, respectively.

Doppler evaluation of adenomyosis usually does not add to the diagnosis because the amount of vascularity is variable and nonspecific.

Differential Diagnosis
If the area of adenomyosis is focal, it may be confused with a fibroid or a polyp if it projects into the endometrial cavity. Because of the lucencies and heterogeneities in the myometrium, uterine malignancy (though very rare) is sometimes considered. The clue to the correct diagnosis is the asymmetry of the width of the myometrium comparing the posterior to the anterior aspect on longitudinal view as well as the shaggy appearance of the endometrial echo in a patient with chronic pain and abnormal bleeding.

Clinical Aspects and Recommendations
Historically, heavy menstrual bleeding (menorrhagia) and painful menstruation (dysmenorrhea) are the major symptoms of adenomyosis and are said to occur in approximately 60% and 25% of women, respectively. It has also been implicated in some cases of chronic pelvic pain. In the past, symptoms typically developed in women in the fourth and fifth decade of life (perimenopausally); however, this probably reflects the fact that in the past the diagnosis of adenomyosis historically was made at the time of hysterectomy and not with sophisticated

imaging techniques as are currently available. In fact the obvious presence of endometrial glands and stroma contained within the myometrium in a large number of asymptomatic women should cause clinicians to rethink whether adenomyosis is truly a "disease" or whether in some cases it may be co-existing and not causal of the patient's symptoms. The exact percentage of patients who will have classic findings of adenomyosis on sophisticated ultrasound studies and yet be totally asymptomatic is unknown.

When present, the menorrhagia is probably related to the increased endometrial surface area of the enlarged uterus. Dysmenorrhea may be caused by the cyclic bleeding and swelling of the endometrial tissue confined within the myometrium.

Definitive treatment for adenomyosis is hysterectomy. Because disease is confined to the uterus, ovarian conservation can be considered unless there are other reasons for their removal. As there is no true plane separating the adenomyotic tissue from normal myometrium, surgical excision as in myomectomy is not appropriate. Various medical (nonsurgical) approaches have been employed, including oral contraceptive pills for treatment of the dysmenorrhea and menorrhagia, progestin only therapy, and more recently levonorgestrel-releasing intrauterine devices (IUDs).

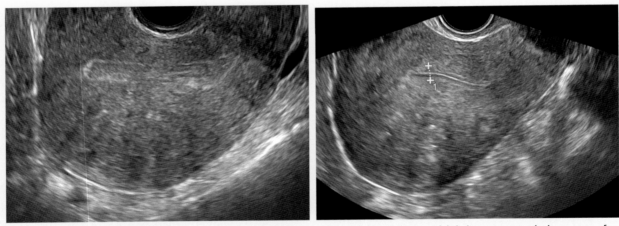

Figure A1-1   Two different patients. Typical appearance of the myometrium, which is asymmetric because of adenomyosis. Note that the endometrial echo is closer to the anterior than the posterior wall of the uterus.

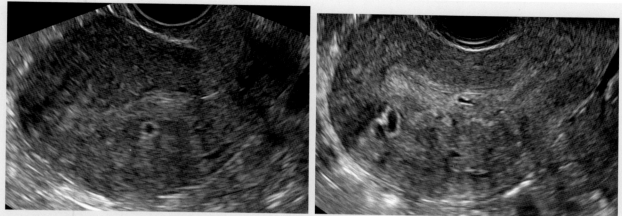

Figure A1-2   Heterogeneous myometrium containing small echolucencies, typical of adenomyosis (two different patients).

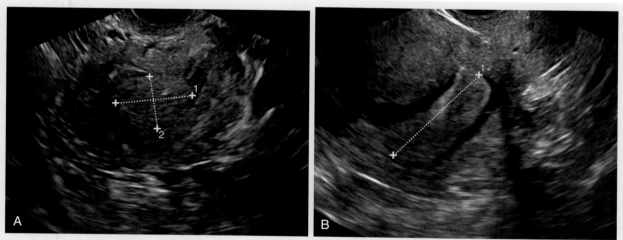

Figure A1-3   Adenomyoma projecting into the endometrial cavity from a broad base within the myometrium.
A shows the mass as ill-defined within the cavity, worrisome for a malignancy, especially in a postmenopausal patient.
B from the same patient shows the sonohysterogram with saline outlining the adenomyoma diagnosed by pathology.

A

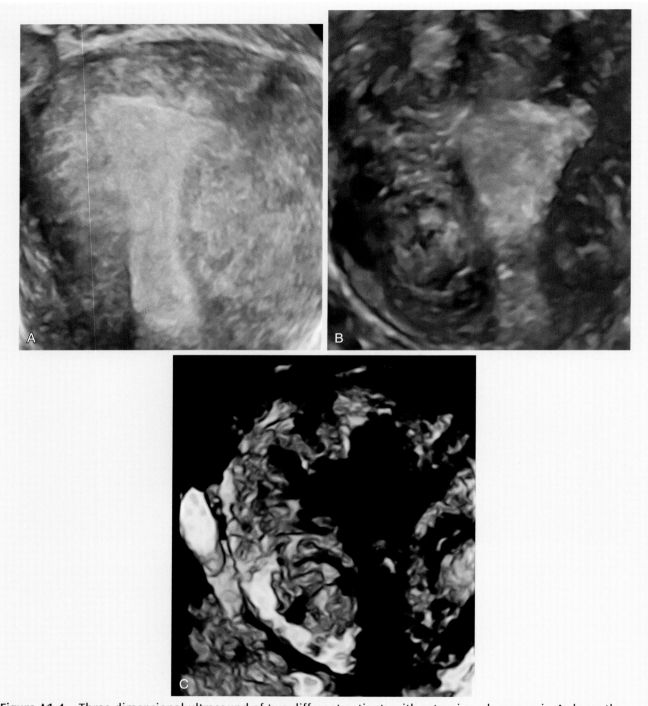

Figure A1-4   Three-dimensional ultrasound of two different patients with extensive adenomyosis. **A** shows the reconstructed coronal view of the uterus with a fuzzy, ill-defined junction and linear echogenicities emanating out from the edges of the endometrium. **B** shows a different patient with adenomyosis and a right-sided fibroid demonstrating similar echolucencies. **C** (same patient as **B**) shows the inverse mode of the 3-D image that accentuates the lack of a clear border at the junction of the endometrium and myometrium.

Suggested Reading

Bocca SM, Oehninger S, Stadtmauer L, Agard J, Duran EH, Sarhan A, Horton S, Abuhamad AZ. A study of the cost, accuracy, and benefits of 3-dimensional sonography compared with hysterosalpingography in women with uterine abnormalities. *J Ultrasound Med.* 2012;31:81-85.

Champaneria R, Abedin P, Daniels J, Balogun M, Khan KS. Ultrasound scan and magnetic resonance imaging for the diagnosis of adenomyosis: systematic review comparing test accuracy. *Acta Obstet Gynecol Scand.* 2010;89:1374-1384.

Exacoustos C, Brienza L, Di Giovanni A, Szabolcs B, Romanini ME, Zupi E, Arduini D. Adenomyosis three-dimensional sonographic findings of the junctional zone and correlation with histology. *Ultrasound Obstet Gynecol.* 2011;37:471-479.

Maheshwari A, Gurunath S, Fatima F, Bhattacharya S. Adenomyosis and subfertility: a systematic review of prevalence, diagnosis, treatment and fertility outcomes. *Hum Reprod Update.* 2012;18:374-392.

Valentini AL, Speca S, Gui B, Soglia G, Miccò M, Bonomo L. Adenomyosis: from the sign to the diagnosis. Imaging, diagnostic pitfalls and differential diagnosis: a pictorial review. *Radiol Med.* 2011;116:1267-1287.

Wéry O, Thille A, Gaspard U, van den Brule F. Adenomyosis: update on a frequent but difficult diagnosis. *J Gynecol Obstet Biol Reprod.* 2005;34:633-648.

A Adhesions (Peritoneal Inclusion Cyst)

Synonyms/Description
Benign adhesions trapping fluid

Etiology
Peritoneal inclusion cysts develop from peritoneal adhesions trapping fluid, often generated from an active ovary. The normal peritoneum absorbs fluid regularly. When the peritoneum is injured, as can occur with surgery, infection, or endometriosis, normal fluid absorption is hampered. This results in fluid accumulation within adhesions or peritoneal inclusion cysts. Reportedly at least 70% of all patients with peritoneal inclusion cysts in one study had a known prior peritoneal insult.

Ultrasound Findings
Peritoneal inclusion cysts are multilocular, cystic masses that conform to the shape of the peritoneum and surrounding organs. They appear as multicystic, septate adnexal or cul-de-sac masses that can be small or attain large sizes. The septations can be thick or thin and can be multiple as the "mass" insinuates itself in the crevices of the pelvic side wall. Often a normal-appearing ovary can be identified embedded along the edges of the mass as the ovary is usually trapped in the web of adhesions but not actually part of the peritoneal inclusion cyst itself.

Differential Diagnosis
Peritoneal inclusion cysts are easily confused with other complex cystic and septate adnexal masses. These include hydrosalpinx, paraovarian cyst, or ovarian neoplasm such as a cystadenoma. In the setting of prior pelvic surgery, the correct diagnosis of peritoneal inclusion cysts can be made, especially if a normal-appearing ovary is seen trapped in the edge of the cyst and the cyst conforms to the shape of the adjacent peritoneal cavity.

Clinical Aspects and Recommendations
Because peritoneal inclusion cysts are virtually always a form of adhesive disease, many of these patients complain of pain, especially with activity such as intercourse, exercise, or bowel movements. This is especially true in those patients whose adhesions are secondary to pelvic inflammatory disease, endometriosis, or possibly, although less likely, previous pelvic surgery. Many peritoneal inclusion cysts, however, are asymptomatic and discovered incidentally during imaging. Because of the variable nature of their sonographic appearance, such "masses" may occasionally appear concerning, and surgical exploration may be undertaken. If such masses are clearly recognized as peritoneal inclusion cysts and are asymptomatic or mildly symptomatic, conservative therapy is appropriate. In most patients with significant pain, surgical correction with lysis of adhesions may be appropriate, although the risk of recurrence is approximately 30% to 50% after surgical treatment.

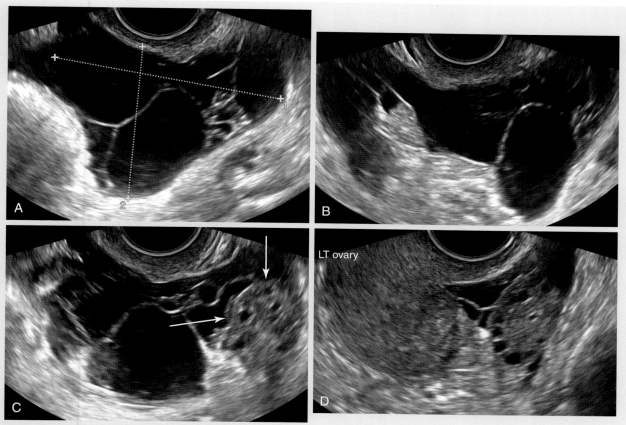

Figure A2-1 **A** and **B** show two views of a left peritoneal inclusion cyst. The top of the ovary is noted along the lateral aspect of the cyst. **C** *(arrows)* and **D** show the ovary in the lateral aspect of the cyst, but showing normal ovarian architecture.

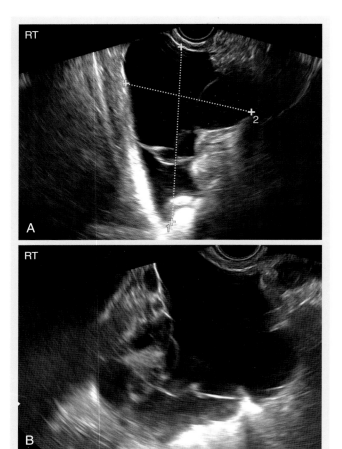

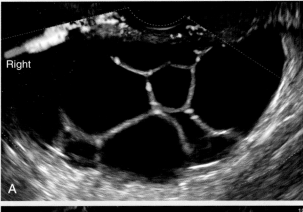

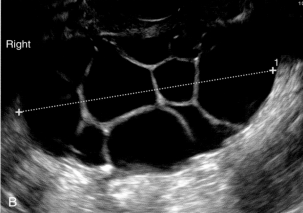

Figure A2-2 Two views of a right peritoneal inclusion cyst. **A** shows the cyst with its typical fine septations. **B** shows the right ovary trapped along the lateral aspect of the cyst.

Figure A2-3 Atypical appearance. **A** shows a multiseptate cystic mass with color flow in the septations, originally thought to be a cystadenoma. **B,** This peritoneal inclusion cyst that was diagnosed at surgery and pathology.

Suggested Reading

Guerriero S, Ajossa S, Mais V, Angiolucci M, Paoletti AM, Melis GB. Role of transvaginal sonography in the diagnosis of peritoneal inclusion cysts. *J Ultrasound Med.* 2004;23:1193-1200.

Jain KA. Imaging of peritoneal inclusion cysts. *Am J Roentgenol.* 2000;174:1559-1563.

Vallerie AM, Lerner JP, Wright JD, Baxi LV. Peritoneal inclusion cysts: a review. *Obstet Gynecol Surv.* 2009; 64:321-334.

Veldhuis WB, Akin O, Goldman D, Mironov S, Mironov O, Soslow RA, Barakat RR, Hricak H. Peritoneal inclusion cysts: clinical characteristics and imaging features. *Eur Radiol.* 2013;23:1167-1174.

Appendiceal Mucocele

A

Synonyms/Description
A mucocele is an appendiceal mass characterized by hypersecretion of mucus contained within the appendix causing dilatation of the lumen.

Etiology
Mucoceles of the appendix are caused by excessive mucous production secondary to retention cyst (simple) (18%), mucosal hyperplasia (20%), mucinous cystadenoma (52% to 84%), or mucinous cystadenocarcinoma (10% to 20%). They occur in males twice as frequently as females and most often in the fifth or sixth decade. The incidence of mucocele of the appendix is 0.2% and 0.3% of all appendectomies.

Ultrasound Findings
Mucocele of the appendix is an elongated tubular mass with a very specific onion-skin texture of the internal structure, giving the appearance of echogenic layers. There is no internal blood flow, and Doppler signal is confined to the outer walls of the mass. Although the mass is usually seen using transvaginal ultrasound, it is also usually visible using a transabdominal approach in the right lower quadrant. The dreaded complication of mucocele rupture or leak is pseudomyxoma peritonei, which appears as diffuse gelatinous ascites.

Differential Diagnosis
Most cases are incidental findings and often misdiagnosed. In women, it is commonly diagnosed as an ovarian or tubal mass. The correct preoperative diagnosis based on imaging studies is made in only 15% to 29% of cases.

The appendix is typically located in the right lower quadrant just cephalad to the right adnexa; therefore it is important to consider an appendiceal etiology for a right lower quadrant tubular mass with or without pelvic pain. Diagnostic possibilities for a complex, right lower quadrant mass include an ovarian etiology, although the tubular appearance of an appendiceal mucocele is more easily confused with a tubal lesion such as a hydrosalpinx, tubo-ovarian abscess, or endometriosis. It is essential to identify the uterus and ovaries separately from the mass to identify a bowel etiology. Once the origin of the mass is suspected to be appendix, the differential diagnosis includes acute inflammation of the appendix (appendicitis), malignancy (adenocarcinoma), mucocele, carcinoid, and appendiceal endometriosis. Other diagnostic possibilities include a colonic mass or mesenteric cyst. The sonographic appearance of the mucocele is very characteristic, even pathognomonic, with the onion-skin texture and nonvascular center of a tubular mass. Other etiologies for an appendiceal mass are almost impossible to distinguish from one another without a history such as acute pain and fever, or endometriosis.

See Bowel Diseases.

Clinical Aspects and Recommendations
Appendiceal mucoceles are symptomatic in about half of cases. The most common symptoms are a palpable mass and abdominal pain. The treatment is appendectomy to prevent rupture and to diagnose any malignant component. If the mucocele is the result of a cystadenocarcinoma and the tumor has spread, more extensive surgery is needed.

The feared complication of this entity is pseudomyxoma peritonei, which results from the dissemination of the mucinous cells because of rupture of the mucocele. This complication is very serious and extremely hard to treat; it can lead to intestinal obstruction and death. Treatment typically involves a combination of surgery for debulking and intraperitoneal chemotherapy. Although the prognosis for appendiceal mucocele without complication is excellent, the 3-year survival of patients with pseudomyxoma peritonei is reportedly 81%.

A

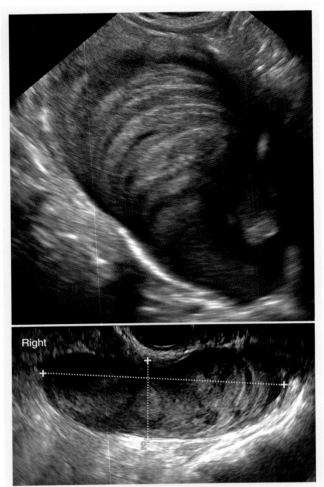

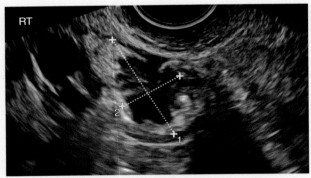

Figure A3-1 Two different patients both suspected of having a tubal lesion but diagnosed by ultrasound to have a mucocele of the appendix. Note the characteristic onion-skin pattern of the linear echoes within both masses revealing the correct diagnosis.

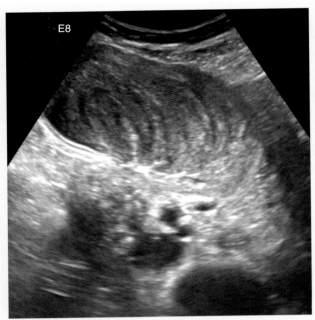

Figure A3-2 Low-grade mucinous cystadenoma. Note the characteristic pattern of linear echoes within the mass.

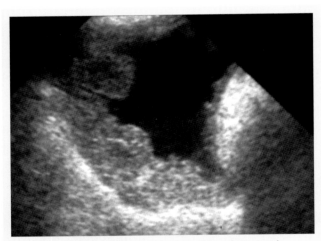

Figure A3-4 Pseudomyxoma peritonei. Note the diffuse involvement of the surfaces of the peritoneal cavity with solid nodular masses.

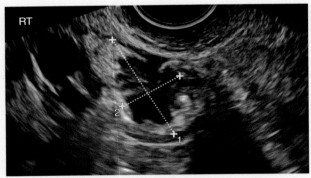

Figure A3-3 Nonspecific appendiceal mass proved to be endometriosis of the appendix.

Videos

Videos 1, 2, and 3 on appendiceal mucocele are available online.

Suggested Reading

Caracappa D, Gullà N, Gentile D, Listorti C, Boselli C, Cirocchi R, Bellezza G, Noya G. Appendiceal mucocele. A case report and literature review. *Ann Ital Chir*. 2011 May-Jun;82(3):239-245.

Dragoumis K, Mikos T, Zafrakas M, Assimakopoulos E, Venizelos I, Demertzidis H, Bontis J. Mucocele of the vermiform appendix with sonographic appearance of an adnexal mass. *Gynecol Obstet Invest*. 2005;59:162-164.

Papoutsis D, Protopappas A, Belitsos P, Sotiropoulou M, Antonakou A, Loutradis D, Antsaklis A. Mucocele of the vermiform appendix misdiagnosed as an adnexal mass on transvaginal sonography. *J Clin Ultrasound*. 2012;40:522-525.

Pickhardt PJ, Levy AD, Rohrmann CA, Kende AI. Primary neoplasms of the appendix: radiologic spectrum of disease with pathologic correlation. *RadioGraphics*. 2003;23:645-662.

Witkamp AJ, de Bree E, Kaag MM, van Slooten GW, van Coevorden F, Zoetmulder FA. Extensive surgical cytoreduction and intraoperative hyperthermic intraperitoneal chemotherapy in patients with pseudomyxoma peritonei. *Br J Surg*. 2001;88: 458-463.

Yabunaka K, Katsuda T, Sanada S, Fukutomi T. Sonographic appearance of the normal appendix in adults. *J Ultrasound Med*. 2007;26:37-43.

A Atrophic Endometrium

Synonyms/Description
Endometrial atrophy

Etiology
Endometrial atrophy is most often the result of postmenopausal status, although it may also occur in premenopausal women with lack of estrogen from other etiologies.

Ultrasound Findings
A very thin endometrial echo is characteristic of atrophic endometrium. This occurs primarily in postmenopausal or anovulatory women. Often the endometrium is so thin it is reflective of sound waves, such that it looks like a continuous line. An atrophic endometrium measures less than 4 mm, but is more commonly 1 to 2 mm in width. In postmenopausal women there can occasionally be a small amount of fluid in the cavity outlining a paper-thin endometrial lining. This is usually transudate associated with cervical stenosis and not associated with pathology.

Differential Diagnosis
If the endometrial lining is very thin in a patient who is hypoestrogenic, the diagnosis is likely to be atrophic endometrium.

Clinical Aspects and Recommendations
Postmenopausal bleeding is often caused by atrophy of the endometrium.

In the absence of estrogen, the functional layer atrophies, leaving only the basalis layer. In patients with postmenopausal bleeding, a workup is necessary to rule out uterine cancer, hyperplasia, and polyps before the cause can be attributed to atrophic endometrium, especially because endometrial cancer can coexist with atrophic endometrium.

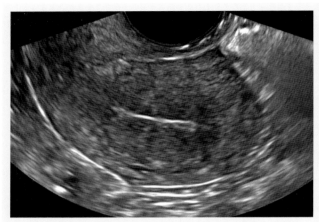

Figure A4-1   Retroverted uterus of a postmenopausal patient with atrophic endometrium. Note the very thin linear endometrial echo.

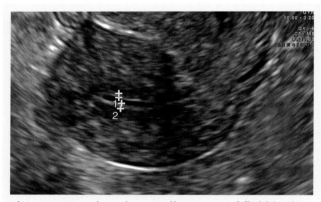

Figure A4-2   There is a small amount of fluid in the endometrial cavity, outlining a very thin endometrium. This finding is normal.

Suggested Reading
Davidson KG, Dubinsky TJ. Ultrasonographic evaluation of the endometrium in postmenopausal vaginal bleeding. *Radiol Clin North Am.* 2003;41: 769-780.

Goldstein SR. Sonography in postmenopausal bleeding. *J Ultrasound Med.* 2012;31:333-336.

Tsai MC, Goldstein SR. Office diagnosis and management of abnormal uterine bleeding. *Clin Obstet Gynecol.* 2012;55(3):635-650.

Bladder Masses

Synonyms/Description
Bladder tumor
Focal bladder lesion

Etiology
Transitional Cell Cancer
In the United States, bladder cancer is reportedly the fourth most common malignancy. The vast majority of bladder neoplasms arise from the epithelium, with urothelial (transitional cell) carcinoma accounting for 90% of cases. Squamous cell carcinoma is rare and accounts for 2% to 15% of bladder cancers. The least common is adenocarcinoma, which may be primary or metastatic to the bladder.

Fibroma
Fibroma (leiomyoma) is the most common benign tumor of the bladder, although it represents only 0.4% of all bladder neoplasms. It is most prevalent among women in the third to fifth decades of life.

Endometriosis
Endometriosis occurs as a fusiform mass in the bladder wall and is covered in the section on endometriosis.

Diffuse Bladder Wall Thickening
Diffuse bladder wall thickening is seen in cases of severe chronic cystitis or in chronic bladder outlet obstruction where the bladder becomes trabeculated (more common in males with large prostates).

Findings Specifically Related to the Ureteral Orifice

- Ureterocele
- Ureteral reimplantation site
- Stone at the ureteropelvic junction (UPJ) with edema of ureteral orifice

Urethral Diverticula
Urethral diverticula occur just under the bladder along the urethra. They can be quite painful, especially when the patient voids.

Other Bladder Masses
There are many benign tumors such as paraganglioma, plasmacytoma, hemangioma, neurofibroma, and lipoma that can occasionally (rarely) occur in the bladder. Malignant neoplasms reported in the bladder include rhabdomyosarcoma, leiomyosarcoma, lymphoma, osteosarcoma, and metastatic tumors such as melanoma.

Ultrasound Findings
Bladder masses are typically located in the bladder wall. Because these arise from the submucosal portion of the bladder wall, they typically appear as smooth intramural lesions. Transitional cell carcinoma is a focal mucosal lesion, which is fungating and extends into the lumen of the bladder with an irregular surface. Color Doppler usually reveals abundant blood flow, as with other pelvic malignancies. Bladder wall lesions are typically fusiform with an intact mucosal surface and focally widen the wall of the bladder. Endometriosis of the bladder wall (likely the most common diagnosis in gynecologic patients) has spotty blood flow by Doppler and a smooth inner and outer wall. Lesions involving the ureteral orifice can be cystic, such as ureteroceles (which are usually asymptomatic); in the case of reimplantations, there will be a surgical history.

Urethral diverticula are complex masses along the urethra, just under the bladder (see Vaginal Masses). These may indent the floor of the bladder and be quite painful during the ultrasound. They are best seen by placing the transducer on the perineum and looking cephalad toward the bladder. They are usually cystic with varying amounts of solid area and calcification, depending on chronicity of the lesion.

B

Differential Diagnosis

Mucosal lesions with an irregular surface and protruding into the bladder are usually transitional cell carcinomas. Lesions that are solid and completely contained within the bladder wall may be endometriosis (fusiform with little detectable blood flow) or fibroma (rounded and ball-like) versus other rare solid rounded tumors.

If the bladder wall is diffusely abnormal and thickened, etiologies may include long-standing bladder dysfunction or obstruction or chronic cystitis. It is normal for the bladder wall to appear thickened and trabeculated if the bladder is underfilled.

If the lesion is along the urethra, it is likely to be a urethral diverticulum.

Clinical Aspects and Recommendations

Bladder lesions can cause dysuria, frequency, and hematuria, but often may be asymptomatic. Bladder malignancies typically present with hematuria because of their location in the mucosal layer of the bladder. Pedunculated intraluminal masses may lead to obstruction of urine flow or inability to completely empty the bladder. If a bladder mass arises in proximity to one of the ureters, it can obstruct the ureter, thus presenting with flank pain and hydronephrosis. Lesions that develop outside the wall of the bladder not impinging on the lumen may remain asymptomatic for a long time. There are no general management recommendations because this depends on the type of lesion diagnosed.

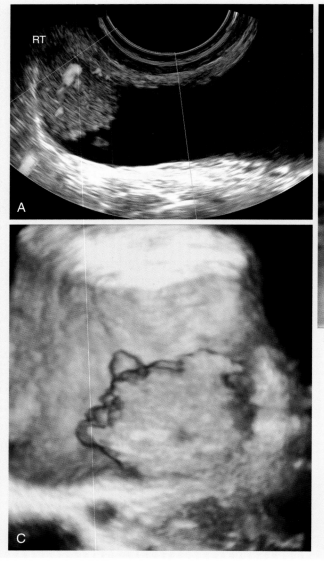

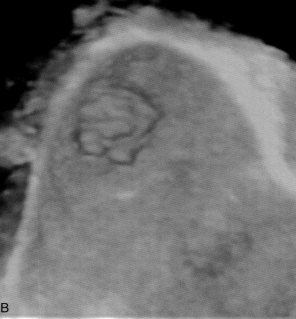

Figure B1-1 Transitional carcinoma of the bladder. **A,** A 2-D view with color Doppler showing abundant vascularity. **B and C,** The same tumor using 3-D surface ultrasound. Note the fungating mucosal surface lesion typical of bladder carcinoma.

B

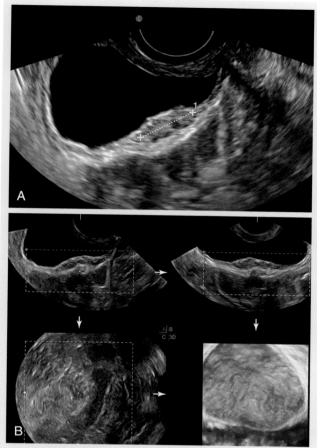

Figure B1-2 A, Fusiform bladder wall mass *(calipers)* in a patient with endometriosis. **B,** The 3-D volume view of the bladder wall mass, showing a smooth mucosal surface.

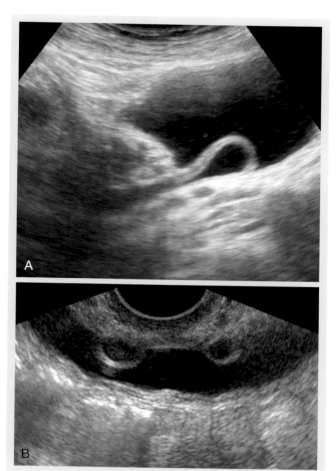

Figure B1-3 Ureterocele. **A,** A longitudinal view of the ureterocele implant into the bladder. **B,** The patient has bilateral ureteroceles.

B

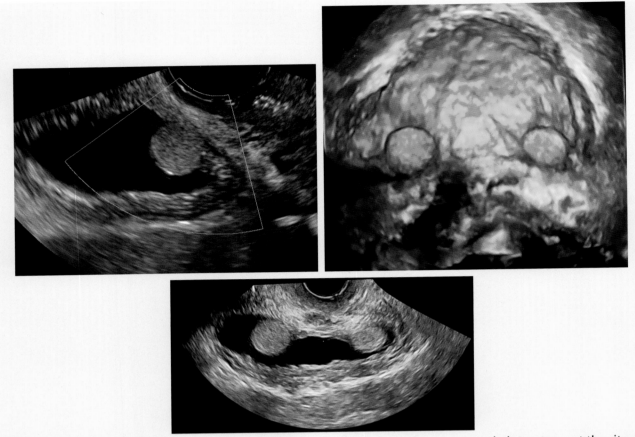

Figure B1-4 Patient with surgically reimplanted ureters. Note the homogeneous rounded structures at the site of reimplantation, 2-D and 3-D.

B

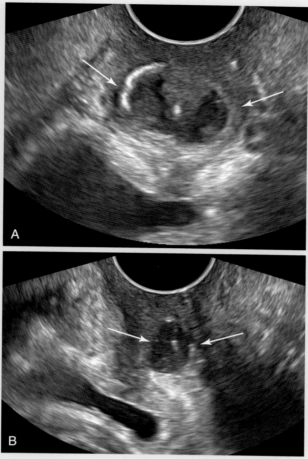

Figure B1-5   Urethral diverticulum *(arrows)*. **A,** Note the complex mass, partly calcified, indenting the floor of the bladder. **B,** The long axis view of the mass alongside the urethra.

B

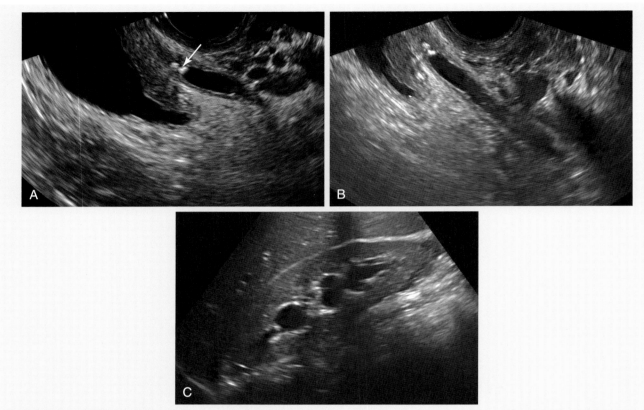

Figure B1-6   A and B, Two small stones stuck in the distal end of the ureter. **C,** The associated hydronephrosis.

Suggested Reading

Fasih N, Prasad Shanbhogue AK, Macdonald DB, Fraser-Hill MA, Papadatos D, Kielar AZ, Doherty GP, Walsh C, McInnes M, Atri M. Leiomyomas beyond the uterus: unusual locations, rare manifestations. *Radiographics.* 2008;28:1931-1948. Review.

Kocakoc E, Kiris A, Orhan I, Poyraz AK, Artas H, Firdolas F. Detection of bladder tumors with 3-dimensional sonography and virtual sonographic cystoscopy. *J Ultrasound Med.* 2008;27:45-53.

Wong-You-Cheong JJ, Woodward PJ, Manning MA, Davis CJ. From the archives of the AFIP: inflammatory and nonneoplastic bladder masses: radiologic-pathologic correlation. *Radiographics.* 2006;26:1847-1868. Review.

Wong-You-Cheong JJ, Woodward PJ, Manning MA, Sesterhenn IA. From the archives of the AFIP: neoplasms of the urinary bladder: radiologic-pathologic correlation. *Radiographics.* 2006;26:553-580. Review.

Borderline Ovarian Tumor

Synonyms/Description
Tumor of low malignant potential (LMP tumor)

Etiology
Ten to fifteen percent of epithelial ovarian tumors are considered borderline malignancies. They tend to occur in women in their forties and fifties, younger than those with frankly invasive tumors, and they are not thought to be related to hereditary breast/ovarian cancer syndromes. These tumors are stage I at diagnosis in more than 90% of patients, have infrequent recurrence, and an excellent prognosis. The survival rates for stage I and stage III are close to 100% and 80% to 90%, respectively. The survival is good even in patients who have developed peritoneal spread. Just more than half are serous, with the rest being mucinous and occasional mixed intestinal cell or endometrioid types. The mucinous tumors tend to be unilateral and are most often of the intestinal type, with a minority being of the endocervical type. Serous tumors have a higher incidence of bilaterality.

Ultrasound Findings
The typical ultrasound appearance of a borderline ovarian cancer is a complex cystic mass with septations, nodularity/papillations, and irregular walls. Flow is typically identified in the solid areas, although not so much flow nor so many irregular vessels as are usually seen in invasive cancers. This difference is neither sufficient nor reliable enough to differentiate invasive from borderline tumors accurately sonographically.

In a study of 113 borderline ovarian tumors, the mucinous tumors of the intestinal type tended to be the largest compared with those of the cervical type or serous lesions. The serous and the mucinous endocervical type of tumors also tended to have a higher number of papillary excrescences and a lower percentage of multilocular lesions when compared with the intestinal type. Solid tumors were found only among the serous tumors.

Differential Diagnosis
The sonographic appearance of borderline tumors is often similar to that of invasive cancers. Other diagnostic possibilities include a decidualized endometrioma in a pregnant woman (see Endometriosis) or a cystadenofibroma. Typically the cystadenofibromas and benign cystadenomas have smaller areas of nodularity with little if any blood flow within the nodule or septae.

Clinical Aspects and Recommendations
The vast majority of mucinous borderline tumors are stage I, with typically benign behavior. On the other hand, the less common endocervical type of mucinous tumor has a worse prognosis, presenting with invasive implants more frequently and recurring more often than the intestinal type. Serous borderline tumors are stage I at presentation in 65% to 70% of cases with a 5-year survival of 95% when there are noninvasive implants and 66% in patients with invasive implants.

The prognosis of patients with borderline ovarian tumors is largely based on the presence of invasive peritoneal implants or residual disease after surgery.

Treatment is surgical removal as well as staging. In patients who have not completed child bearing, the uterus and contralateral ovary may be preserved.

Increasingly in stage I disease, ovarian cystectomy only and close observation are being advocated for those who have not completed child bearing.

B

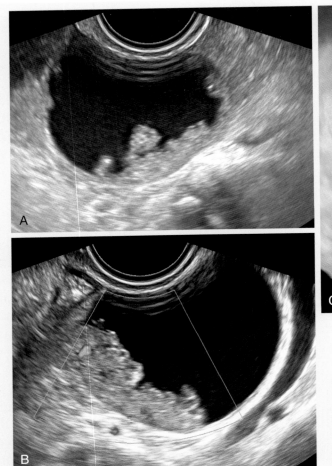

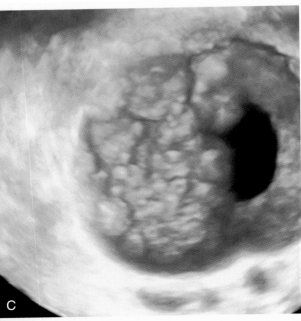

Figure B2-1 A papillary serous cystadenoma with irregular nodularity. **A,** The lateral side of the mass. **B,** The medial side with thicker nodularity. Note the modest blood flow in the solid areas, less than would be expected in a more aggressive tumor. **C,** A 3-D image of the surface texture of the inner aspect of the tumor.

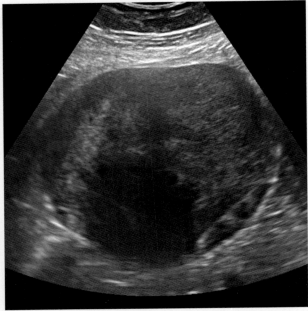

Figure B2-2 A mucinous borderline tumor. Note the abundant solid portions and unilocular and large lesion.

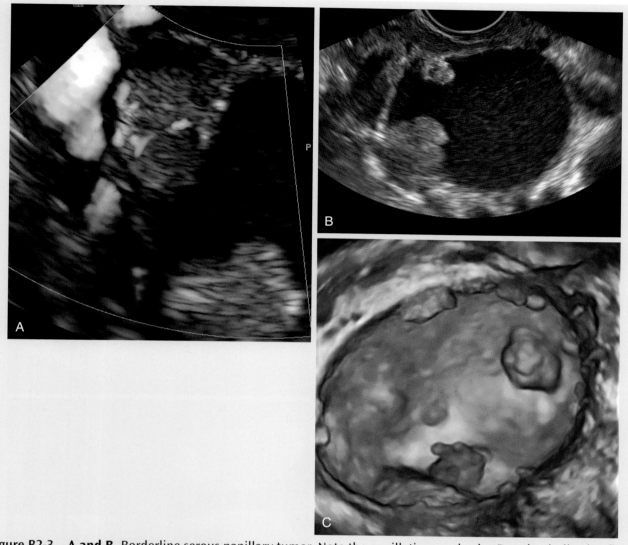

Figure B2-3 A and B, Borderline serous papillary tumor. Note the papillations and color Doppler, indicating flow in the solid areas. **C,** The papillations using 3-D surface imaging.

B

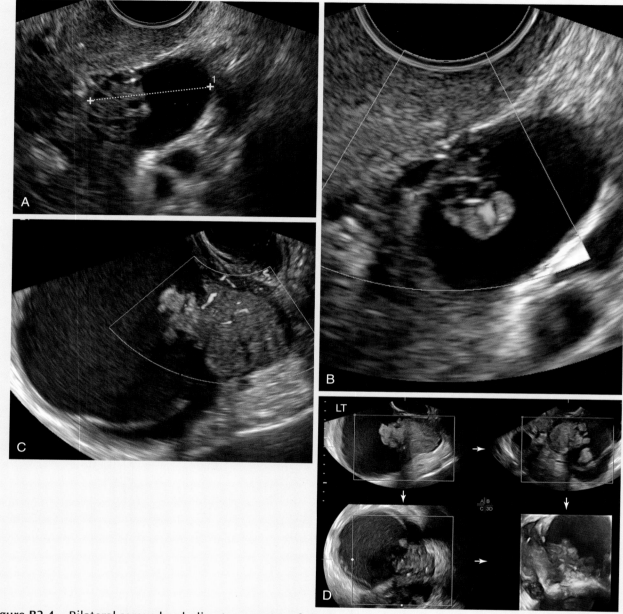

Figure B2-4 Bilateral serous borderline tumors. **A and B,** The left ovarian mass with the small lesion containing a single vascular nodule. **C,** The right ovarian mass is larger, with low-level echoes and a large vascular nodule. **D,** A 3-D volume illustrating the surface of the nodularity.

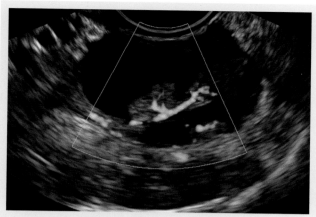

Figure B2-5 Color flow is seen using Doppler in the septation of this borderline tumor.

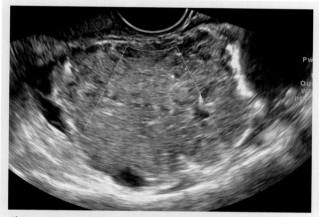

Figure B2-6 The unusually solid appearance of a borderline tumor, mimicking an invasive cancer.

Suggested Reading

Behtash N, Modares M, Abolhasani M, Ghaem-maghami F, Mousavi M, Yarandi F, Hanjani P. Borderline ovarian tumours: clinical analysis of 38 cases. *J Obstet Gynaecol.* 2004;24:157-160.

Fruscella E, Testa AC, Ferrandina G, De Smet F, Van Holsbeke C, Scambia G, Zannoni FG, Ludovisi M. Ultrasound features of different histopathological subtypes of borderline ovarian tumors. *Ultrasound Obstet Gynecol.* 2005;26:644-650.

Morice P, Uzan C, Fauvet R, Gouy S, Duvillard P, Darai E. Borderline ovarian tumour: pathological diagnostic dilemma and risk factors for invasive or lethal recurrence. *Lancet Oncol.* 2012;13:103-115.

Tropé CG, Kaern J, Davidson B. Borderline ovarian tumours. *Best Pract Res Clin Obstet Gynaecol.* 2012;26:325-336.

B

Bowel Diseases

Synonyms/Description

Pelvic masses related to bowel such as appendicitis, endometriosis, colon cancer, Crohn's disease, ulcerative colitis, diverticulitis, lymphoma, sarcoma, or other bowel-specific diseases identified on a pelvic ultrasound

Etiology

There are multiple etiologies in this grouping of bowel diseases. The etiologies range from inflammatory/infectious such as appendicitis, inflammatory bowel diseases, and diverticulitis to neoplasms such as lymphomas, carcinomas, and sarcomas.

In the small bowel, neuroendocrine tumors, adenocarcinomas, sarcomas, lymphomas, and miscellaneous tumors comprise 36.5%, 30.9%, 10.0%, 18.7%, and 3.9% of malignancies, respectively. In the appendix, neuroendocrine tumors, adenocarcinomas, sarcomas, lymphomas, and miscellaneous tumors comprise 31.7%, 65.4%, greater than 1%, 1.7%, and 1.1% of malignancies, respectively. Colon tumors include mostly adenocarcinomas (93.0%), whereas sarcomas and lymphomas are relatively rare.

These entities are briefly discussed in terms of ultrasound findings because they may be encountered during a sonographic gynecologic exam. For more detailed information about any of these lesions, please refer to the suggested reading.

Ultrasound Findings

Diseases of the bowel are detectable and can be accurately diagnosed using ultrasound. Typically the sonographic evaluation of bowel abnormalities includes the appearance of the bowel wall, amount and quality of peristalsis, reaction to manual compression using the transducer, and relative "stiffness" of the bowel loop. Also there may be a nonspecific mass, which is difficult to distinguish from adnexal or uterine masses. It is crucial to identify the uterus and ovaries separate from the mass to correctly diagnose it as a bowel problem.

Endometriosis

Endometriosis of the rectosigmoid colon is covered in the section on endometriosis.

Appendicitis

The typical ultrasound findings include a distended, noncompressible tubular mass, greater than 7 mm in diameter and with relatively cystic center suggesting bowel. In the transverse view, the abnormal appendix often appears as a double ring indicating the swollen wall. Gentle compression will displace normal loops of bowel to better demonstrate the inflamed appendix, although the compression is usually uncomfortable for the patient. There can also be inflammation of the adjacent omental fat with a very echogenic characteristic appearance, sometimes with shadowing from an appendicolith. The sensitivity for ultrasound compared with computed tomography to diagnose appendicitis is 75% versus 90%, and the specificity is 86% versus 100%. Ultrasound is often the only imaging needed to make the diagnosis.

Inflammatory Bowel Diseases

These include Crohn's disease and ulcerative colitis, which typically produce a diffuse thickening of a segment of bowel wall, with reduced peristalsis and a "stiff-looking," relatively straight segment of bowel. There is usually a loss of the normal striated gut appearance because of the disease involving multiple layers of the bowel wall. Ulcerative colitis is found mostly in the rectum and rectosigmoid, whereas Crohn's is typically seen in the distal ileum.

Diverticulitis

When a diverticulum becomes inflamed, it appears sonographically as a segmental area of thickened bowel wall with an inflamed out-pouching (diverticulum) and inflamed surrounding pericolic fat. Diverticulitis can also result in an abscess that can be seen sonographically. The bowel wall thickening is usually asymmetric but retains its normal three layers, thus differentiating it from the appearance of inflammatory bowel disease.

Duplication Cyst

Bowel duplication cysts are rare congenital anomalies that may be asymptomatic for much of a person's life. However, when these undergo hemorrhage, infection, or torsion, the symptoms are similar to appendicitis or ovarian torsion. Sonographically, when these cysts are symptomatic, they will show internal hemorrhage and appear similar to an endometrioma.

Lymphoma

Lymphomas of the bowel wall are typically B-cell tumors and usually involve the small intestine in the region of the distal ileum. The ultrasound appearance is that of a bulky circumferential irregular wall thickening with occasional dilation of the bowel and lymph node enlargement.

Colon Cancer

Adenocarcinoma is the most common malignant tumor of the colon. The ultrasound appearance is that of a hypoechoic mass with many tiny echogenic septations, some areas of calcification, and a bubbly or airy texture. In many cases, the original loop of colon affected is difficult to see sonographically and often the mass is not initially attributed to the bowel.

Gastrointestinal Stromal Tumor

These are a group of mesenchymal sarcomas that arise typically from the muscularis mucosa of the bowel wall and are therefore submucosal. Gastrointestinal stromal tumors (GISTs) are homogeneous soft-tissue solid masses that may be small or grow into a large necrotic, heterogeneous mass. They are usually malignant tumors that can metastasize to the liver.

Differential Diagnosis

The main differential diagnosis for a tender mass in the right lower quadrant includes appendicitis as well as many gynecologic etiologies such as hydrosalpinx, hemorrhagic cyst, or degenerating fibroid. It is important to view the mass transabdominally as well as transvaginally to get a better sense of its location. As previously discussed, identifying the uterus and ovaries separately from the mass is essential to making the correct diagnosis.

A thickened loop of bowel suggests a more diffuse diagnosis such as lymphoma or chronic inflammatory disease. A focal area of bowel wall nodularity or thickening may indicate an endometriotic implant or diverticulitis. (A careful history may help differentiate these diagnoses.) A solitary mass separate from the uterus or ovaries may represent a bowel tumor such as a leiomyoma, sarcoma, or adenocarcinoma. A cyst separate from the ovary or tube may represent a bowel duplication cyst, although these can be confused with endometriomas.

Clinical Aspects and Recommendations

Ultrasound should be the first test done in patients suspected of having appendicitis and is often sufficient to make an accurate diagnosis. In many cases of bowel malignancy or chronic inflammatory disease, other imaging modalities and procedures are necessary to arrive at the correct diagnosis, and the treatment and prognosis depend on the final diagnosis. However, ultrasound may be the entry point at which patients with various bowel problems enter the medical care system, and it is important to keep these diagnoses in mind when performing pelvic ultrasound.

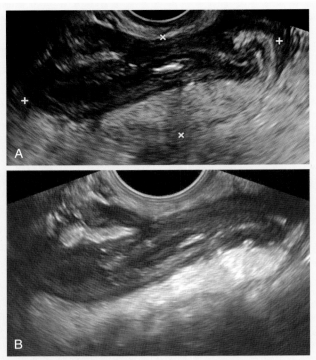

Figure B3-1   A and B, Transvaginal view of acute appendicitis (longitudinal and transverse views). The calipers show the distended thick-walled appendix with echogenic surrounding edema. This was misdiagnosed as a tubal abscess.

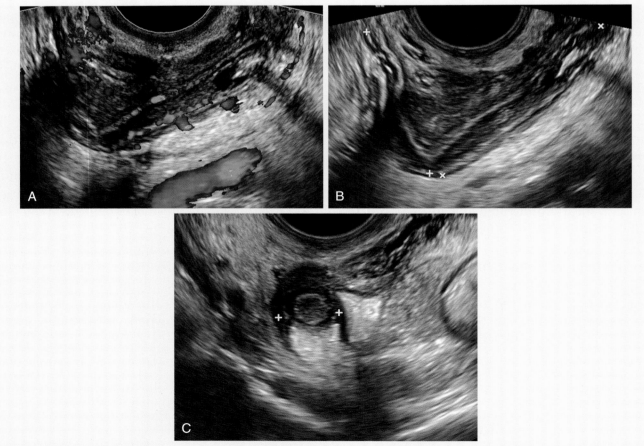

Figure B3-2   A, B, and C, Same case as Figure B3-1 after a course of antibiotic and after the correct diagnosis of appendicitis had been made.

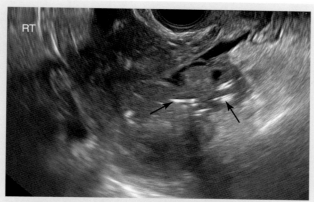

Figure B3-3 Appendiceal abscess, seen transvaginally, with characteristic linear echogenicities with shadowing consistent with air pockets.

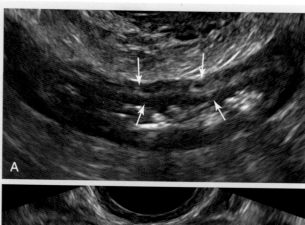

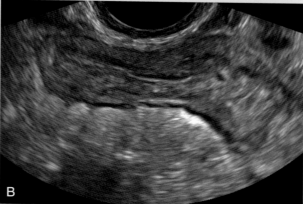

Figure B3-5 **A and B,** Two different patients, both with Crohn's disease. Note the diffuse bowel wall thickening in a relatively straight loop of bowel, with loss of architecture of the wall layers.

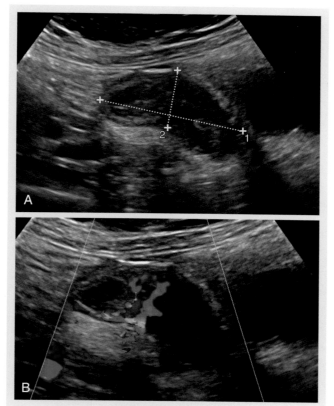

Figure B3-4 **A and B,** Enlarged appendix later diagnosed as adenocarcinoma of the appendix.

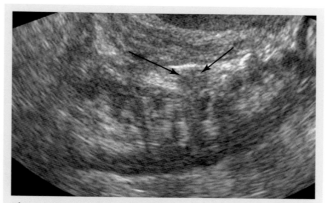

Figure B3-6 Multiple diverticula in a loop of colon. Note the smooth posterior wall compared with the multiple outpouchings *(arrows)* of the anterior wall.

B

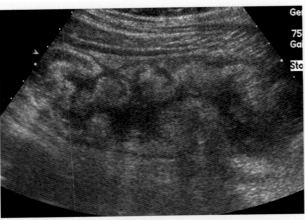

Figure B3-7   Lymphoma. Note the marked thickening of the bowel wall with complete loss of normal architecture. The appearance is that of a diffuse and global process involving a long segment of bowel.

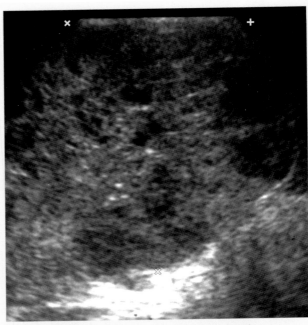

Figure B3-9   Colon cancer. Note the complex mass with multiple bright areas and irregular septations. This is a characteristic bubbly or airy texture often seen with this tumor.

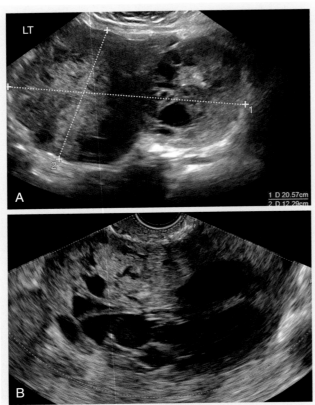

Figure B3-8   A and B, Gastrointestinal stromal sarcoma (GIST tumor). Note the large 20-cm tumor, mostly solid but with a few cystic spaces. **B** shows relatively little internal blood flow because of necrotic spaces.

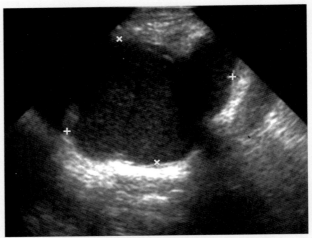

Figure B3-10   Rectal duplication cyst, originally mistaken for an endometrioma in a patient presenting with pelvic pain.

Videos

Video 1 on bowel-related masses is available online.

Suggested Reading

Ackerman SJ, Irshad A, Anis M. Ultrasound for pelvic pain. II: Nongynecologic causes. *Obstet Gynecol Clin North Am.* 2011;38:69-83.

Gustafsson BI, Siddique L, Chan A, Dong M, Drozdov I, Kidd M, Modlin IM. Uncommon cancers of the small intestine, appendix and colon: an analysis of SEER 1973-2004, and current diagnosis and therapy. *Int J Oncol.* 2008;33:1121-1131.

Hughes JA, Cook JV, Said A, Chong SK, Towu E, Reidy J. Gastrointestinal stromal tumour of the duodenum in a 7-year-old boy. *Pediatr Radiol.* 2004;34:1024-1027.

Lee NK, Kim S, Kim GH, Jeon TY, Kim DH, Jang HJ, Park DY. Hypervascular subepithelial gastrointestinal masses: CT-pathologic correlation. *RadioGraphics.* 2010;30:1915-1934.

Linam LE, Munden M. Sonography as the first line of evaluation in children with suspected acute appendicitis. *J Ultrasound Med.* 2012;31:1153-1157.

Maturen KE, Wasnik AP, Kamaya A, Dillman JR, Kaza RK, Pandya A, Maheshwary RK. Ultrasound imaging of bowel pathology: technique and keys to diagnosis in the acute abdomen. *AJR.* 2011;197:1067-1075.

O'Malley ME, Wilson SR. Ultrasound of gastrointestinal tract abnormalities with CT correlation. *RadioGraphics.* 2003;23:59-72.

B

Brenner Tumor

B

Synonyms/Description
Transitional cell tumor of the ovary
Typically asymptomatic, rare, benign ovarian tumor

Etiology
These tumors account for approximately 3.2% of ovarian epithelial neoplasms and typically occur in the fourth to sixth decades of life. They belong to the combined surface epithelial-stromal group of tumors, although they have been described as having similar histologic appearance to transitional cell tumors of the urothelium.

Ultrasound Findings
These masses are typically solid, hypoechoic, frequently contain some calcifications, and have minimal detectable color Doppler flow. Approximately 25% of the time, there is a cystic component indicating the possible presence of a co-existent cystic epithelial neoplasm, such as a serous or mucinous cystadenoma. These cystic components can have solid papillations, and they may be malignant (about 15% of cases).

Differential Diagnosis
Most Brenner tumors appear similar sonographically to other solid ovarian masses such as fibromas-thecomas, and can be mistaken for pedunculated fibroids. Those with complex cystic components are indistinguishable from serous and mucinous cystadenoma/cystadenocarcinoma, or endometrioid carcinoma.

Clinical Aspects and Recommendations
These are rare ovarian masses that are typically asymptomatic. Management depends on the type of mass, which can be benign, proliferative, or (rarely) malignant. If intervention is indicated, surgical management is undertaken.

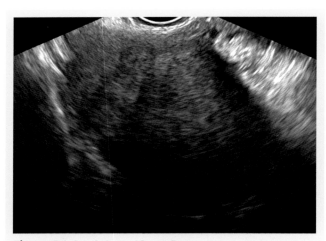

Figure B4-1 A 1- to 10-cm Brenner tumor masquerading as a pedunculated fibroid. Note the heterogeneous texture of the tumor with linear shadows similar to fibromas.

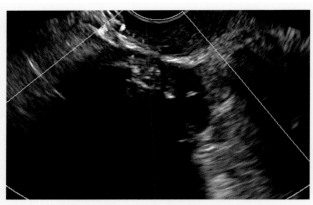

Figure B4-2 Longitudinal view of a Brenner tumor with extensive calcification and shadowing.

Suggested Reading

Athey PA, Siegel MF. Sonographic features of Brenner tumor of the ovary. *J Ultrasound Med.* 1987;6: 367-372.

Dierickx I, Valentin L, Van Holsbeke C, Jacomen G, Lissoni AA, Licameli A, Testa A, Bourne T, Timmerman D. Imaging in gynecological disease (7): clinical and ultrasound features of Brenner tumors of the ovary. *Ultrasound Obstet Gynecol.* 2012;40: 706-713.

Green GE, Mortele KJ, Glickman JN, Benson CB. Brenner tumors of the ovary: sonographic and computed tomographic imaging features. *J Ultrasound Med.* 2006;25:1245-1251.

Hermanns B, Faridi A, Rath W, Füzesi L, Schröder W. Differential diagnosis, prognostic factors, and clinical treatment of proliferative Brenner tumor of the ovary. *Ultrastruct Pathol.* 2000;24:191-196.

Hiroi H, Osuga Y, Tarumoto Y, Shimokama T, Yano T, Yokota H, Taketani Y. A case of estrogen-producing Brenner tumor with a stromal component as a potential source for estrogen. *Oncology.* 2002;63:201-204.

B

Cervical Masses

C

Synonyms/Description
None

Etiology
Cervical cancer accounts for the majority of cervical malignancies and is second to breast cancer in incidence worldwide. Approximately 85% to 95% of cervical cancers are squamous cell carcinomas and develop at the squamous-columnar junction.

Adenocarcinomas represent only 5% of cervical cancers and arise from glandular cells found in the endocervical canal. Squamous cell lesions of the cervix are typically detected early using conventional cytologic screening methods (Pap test) because they are easy to sample. The majority of endocervical glands are deep within the cervical canal, so detection usually occurs at more advanced stages of disease; hence they have a poorer prognosis than squamous cell cancers. The survival for stages I, II, and III cervical adenocarcinoma is 60%, 47%, and 8% compared with 90%, 62%, and 36% for squamous cell carcinoma.

Non-Hodgkin's lymphoma of the cervix is rare, accounting for 1% of all extranodal lymphomas. Clinically it may present as a large lobular vascular solid mass of the cervix. Metastatic disease, such as melanoma and breast, lung, and ovarian cancers, may also involve the cervix.

Malignant mixed Müllerian tumors and leiomyosarcomas occur more frequently in the uterine corpus, but may arise in the cervix in rare cases. Embryonal rhabdomyosarcomas typically occur in the pediatric age group.

Benign masses of the cervix include fibroids and polyps, which are similar in origin and appearance to their counterparts in the uterine corpus. Nabothian cysts are also commonly seen.

Ultrasound Findings
Cervical masses can obstruct the cervical canal and result in a hematometra, which may be the first sonographic sign of a cervical malignancy. Cervical carcinomas, especially squamous, are often subtle or undetectable sonographically as they can be quite small. As they grow, they appear as solid lobulated masses with abundant vascularity. Sarcomas and lymphomas are typically large solid vascular tumors when discovered. The appearance of these malignant tumors is nonspecific, although the excessive and disorganized blood flow within the tumor suggests a malignancy. Epstein and colleagues compared the sonographic characteristics of squamous cell and adenocarcinoma of the cervix. The ultrasound appearances of the tumors were all solid masses; however, 73% of the squamous cell carcinomas were hypoechoic, whereas 68% of the adenocarcinomas were isoechoic ($p = 0.03$). Mixed echogenicity was a nonspecific finding, and Doppler color flow was abundant in almost all the tumors of both types.

Benign masses of the cervix also tend to be solid sonographically, although the blood flow pattern seen with color Doppler tends to be different from that of the cancers. Polyps typically have a single feeding vessel, and are usually echogenic, sometimes containing a cystic center. Fibroids are solid masses with a similar appearance to those in the uterine corpus. They are well circumscribed, with acoustic shadowing, often with a pattern of stripes or swirls caused by these shadows. The blood flow in fibroids is variable although less abundant than in malignant lesions and more peripheral.

Nabothian cysts appear as very smooth and round, cystic, hypoechoic masses without any areas of Doppler color flow, and are extremely common, especially in women with previous pregnancies.

Differential Diagnosis

The differential diagnosis for a cervical mass includes the common entities such as a polyp or fibroid. If the mass is lobulated and highly vascular, a cervical malignancy such as a carcinoma, lymphoma, sarcoma, or metastatic tumor must be considered. A biopsy is necessary to arrive at a definitive diagnosis because these cervical malignancies have a similar sonographic appearance. Transvaginal ultrasound can also be helpful for staging of cervical cancers although MRI, CT, and PET/CT are typically used for these work-ups.

Clinical Aspects and Recommendations

The management of a sonographically detectable cervical mass depends on the etiology. Masses that are hypervascular or that appear atypical should be biopsied. However, simple punch biopsy may be inadequate, especially for tumors arising or metastasizing deep in the cervix. A bulky cervical non-Hodgkin's lymphoma may present as an irregular, palpable, bulky mass, but a punch biopsy will often reveal normal squamous tissue. A cone or excisional biopsy is required in cases in which the initial biopsy does not correlate with the sonographic findings. Management then depends on the diagnosis. Malignancies are treated with multiple modalities, including, but not limited to, surgery, radiation, chemotherapy, and immunotherapy. Asymptomatic fibroids do not typically require treatment, except in cases in which they may affect reproductive outcomes. When indicated, treatment is generally surgical. Cervical polyps often present with spotting and usually can be excised, although dilation and curettage may be required to get the entire stalk removed. Nabothian cysts are not pathologic, and thus no treatment is indicated.

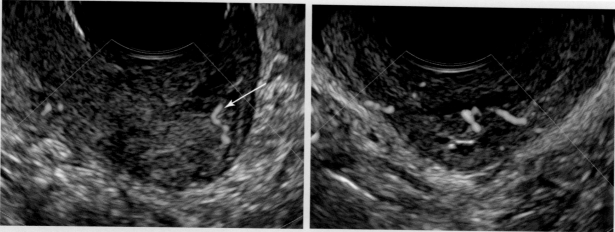

Figure C1-1   Small squamous cell carcinoma of the surface of the cervix, identified by the cluster of blood vessels *(arrow)* on the external os region.

C

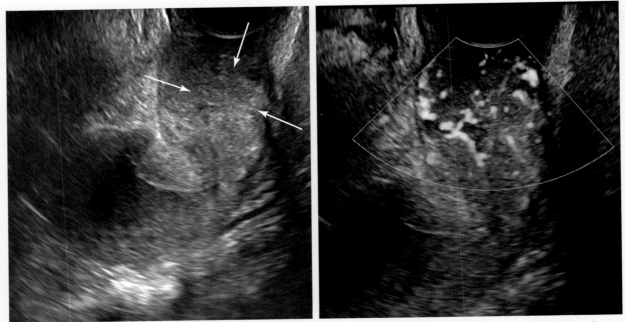

Figure C1-2 Transvaginal view of a large cervical tumor *(arrows)* with abundant blood flow, arising from the endocervical canal and protruding through the cervix. This proved to be an adenocarcinoma of the cervix.

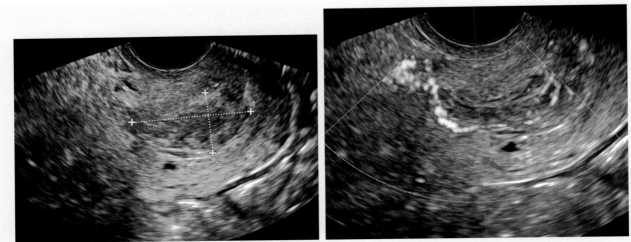

Figure C1-3 Cervical polyp originating from the lower uterine segment and protruding through the cervix. Note the feeding vessel.

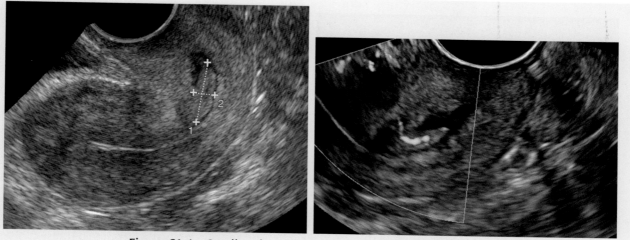

Figure C1-4   Small endocervical polyp with single feeder vessel.

C

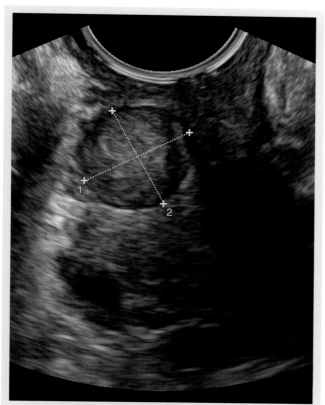

Figure C1-5   Cervical fibroid. Note the round, well-demarcated mass on the side of the cervix.

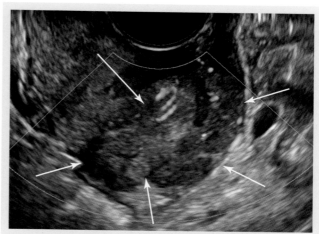

Figure C1-6   Cervical lymphoma. Note the large mass *(arrows)* with modest vascularity surrounding the entire outer aspect of the cervix.

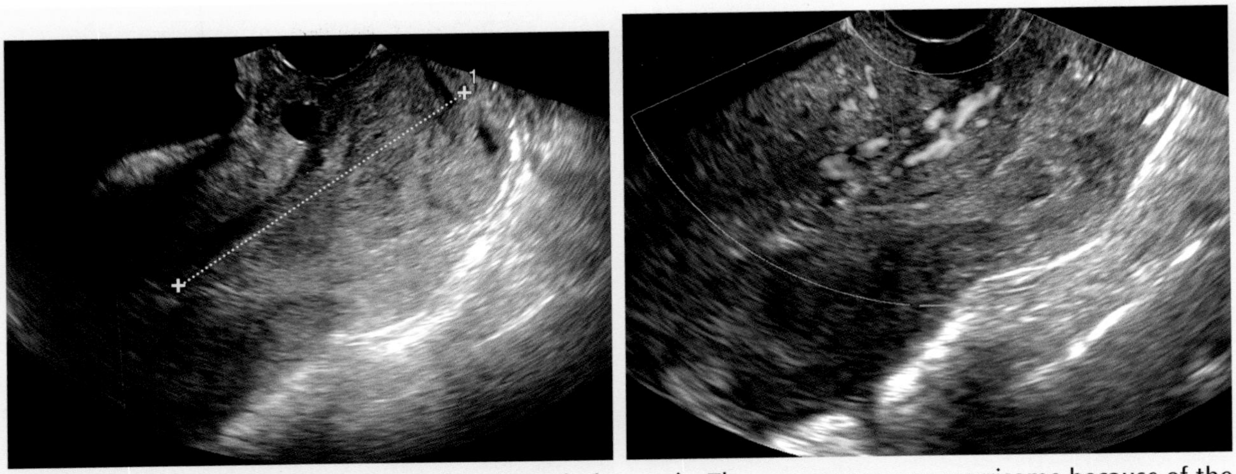

Figure C1-7 Large vascular mass protruding through the cervix. The appearance was worrisome because of the heterogeneity of the mass and the abundant blood flow. This mass proved to be a benign fibroid at surgery.

Suggested Reading

Chan JK, Loizzi V, Magistris A, Hunter MI, Rutgers J, DiSaia PJ, Berman ML. Clinicopathologic features of six cases of primary cervical lymphoma. *Am J Obstet Gynecol.* 2005;193:866-872.

Epstein E, Di Legge A, Måsbäck A, Lindqvist PG, Kannisto P, Testa AC. Sonographic characteristics of squamous cell cancer and adenocarcinoma of the uterine cervix. *Ultrasound Obstet Gynecol.* 2010;36(4): 512-516.

Gaurilcikas A, Vaitkiene D, Cizauskas A, Inciura A, Svedas E, Maciuleviciene R, Di Legge A, Ferrandina G, Testa AC, Valentin L. Early-stage cervical cancer: agreement between ultrasound and histopathological findings with regard to tumor size and extent of local disease. *Ultrasound Obstet Gynecol.* 2011;38(6): 707-715.

Sahdev A. Cervical tumors. *Semin Ultrasound CT MR.* 2010;31(5):399-413.

Semczuk A, Skomra D, Korobowicz E, Balon B, Rechberger T. Primary non-Hodgkin's lymphoma of the uterine cervix mimicking leiomyoma: case report and review of the literature. *Pathol Res Pract.* 2006;202:61-64.

Cesarean Scar Defect

Synonyms/Description
Uterine dehiscence

Etiology
Cesarean sections (C-sections) are performed in the United States at the rate of 20% to 50% of deliveries depending on clinical environment and demographics. The C-section scar is readily visible sonographically in the nonpregnant uterus as a focal narrowing of the anterior lower uterine segment, which becomes more pronounced with increasing number of prior sections. There is often a small myometrial discontinuity within the scar, seen as a triangular fluid collection or "niche," likely representing menstrual blood that pools within the defect. Many patients who have had C-sections complain of intermittent inter-menstrual or prolonged menstrual bleeding. Uppal and colleagues reported that among 71 patients with a history of C-section, 29 (40%) had a sonographically visible fluid-filled defect in the hysterotomy incision, and the presence of such a defect was significantly associated with prolonged periods or intermenstrual spotting. The incidence of abnormal bleeding was more frequent in patients with larger defects, and the size of the defect or niche was directly related to the number of prior C-sections. Wang and colleagues studied 207 patients with C-section scars and also found that those who had multiple C-sections had larger myometrial defects (width and depth) compared with those with only one prior C-section. Patients with retroflexed uteri also had wider defects than those whose uterus was anteflexed.

The myometrial thickness at the C-section scar becomes thinner as the number of C-sections increases; however, there is no established norm for this measurement. The presence of a C-section scar defect and the size of this myometrial niche seem to be better predictors of abnormal bleeding and even risk of uterine dehiscence in subsequent pregnancies.

Ultrasound Findings
The C-section scar defect is a wedge-shaped cystic or hypoechoic area in the anterior lower uterine segment myometrium, directly above the level of the cervix.

Saline distention of the cavity during a sono-hysterogram can further delineate the scar defect, if clinically indicated. This more clearly shows the diverticulum-like outpouching of the endometrial cavity into the thinned, scarred myometrium.

Occasionally if the patient has had a classical C-section, a vertical scar can be seen on the front of the uterus, puckering the length of the body of the uterus (see Figure C2-3).

Rarely the C-section scar can dehisce, resulting in a myometrial defect, bulging anteriorly under the bladder. This cystic mass typically has low-level echoes consistent with unclotted blood that has accumulated during menses (see Figure C2-2).

Differential Diagnosis
The appearance of a C-section scar defect is characteristic and unmistakable. If the scar has ballooned anteriorly and caused a cystic mass in the lower uterine segment, the lesion could be confused with a degenerating fibroid or even a lesion involving the floor of the bladder such as an endometrioma. Most cases of C-section scar defects do not present a diagnostic dilemma.

Clinical Aspects and Recommendations
The presence of a fluid collection in the scar defect is an important finding that may explain abnormal uterine bleeding in some patients. It has also been associated with dysmenorrhea as well as infertility. At this point, most of the research is still focused on the prevalence and conditions associated with C-section scar defects. There are some reports of surgical repair of the defects resulting in improved fertility and resolution of prolonged or intermenstrual bleeding. Given that this is a relatively new, although rapidly increasing diagnostic entity, there are as of yet no standard recommendations.

C

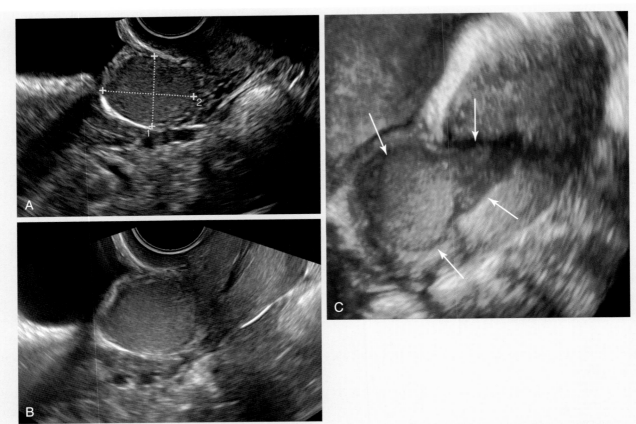

Figure C2-1   Longitudinal view of the normal uterus of a patient with a C-section scar defect. A small amount of fluid outlines the C-section scar defect *(arrow)* in the anterior lower uterine segment where the C-section scar is located. The niche is formed by the puckering of the anterior wall of the uterus, just above the cervix.

Figure C2-2   Large rounded area of dehiscence of a C-section scar ballooning anteriorly and indenting the bladder. **A and B,** Two-dimensional views of the lower uterine segment taken obliquely, showing the mass-like defect between the cervix and bladder. The defect *(calipers)* is filled with low-level echoes indicating unclotted blood. Note the proximity of the defect to the bladder. **C,** A 3-D longitudinal view of the anterior aspect of the uterus, showing the defect *(arrows)* originating from the lower uterine segment and bulging anteriorly at the level of the C-section scar.

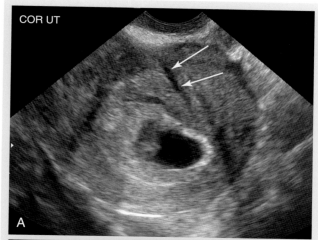

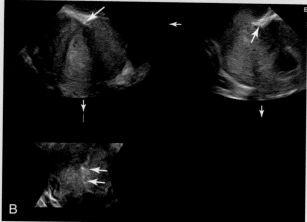

Figure C2-3   Classical C-section scar in a pregnant patient. **A,** Note the puckering of the anterior surface of the entire uterus *(arrows)*. **B,** A 3-D multiplanar reconstruction of the uterus showing the linear vertical scar in three orientations *(arrows)*.

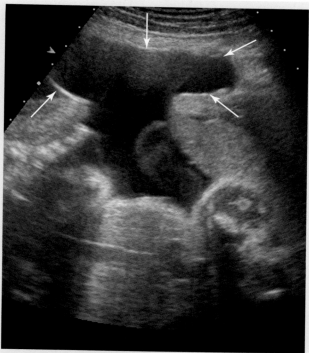

Figure C2-4   Dehiscence of the C-section scar in a pregnant patient with one prior section. The membranes are seen herniating through the defect in the lower uterine segment *(arrows)*.

Suggested Reading

Bujold E, Jastrow N, Simoneau J, Brunet S, Gauthier RJ. Prediction of complete uterine rupture by sonographic evaluation of the lower uterine segment. *Am J Obstet Gynecol.* 2009;201:320.

Jastrow N, Chaillet N, Roberge S, Morency AM, Lacasse Y, Bujold E. Sonographic lower uterine segment thickness and risk of uterine scar defect: a systematic review. *J Obstet Gynaecol Can.* 2010;32:321-327.

Monteagudo A, Carreno C, Timor-Tritsch IE. Saline infusion sonohysterography in nonpregnant women with previous cesarean delivery: the "niche" in the scar. *J Ultrasound Med.* 2001;20:1105-1115.

Naji O, Abdallah Y, Bij De Vaate AJ, Smith A, Pexsters A, Stalder C, Mcindoe A, Ghaem-Maghami S. Standardized approach for imaging and measuring Cesarean section scars using ultrasonography. *Ultrasound Obstet Gynecol.* 2012;39:252-259.

Uppal T, Lanzarone V, Mongelli M. Sonographically detected caesarean section scar defects and menstrual irregularity. *J Obstet Gynaecol.* 2011;31:413-416.

Vikhareva Osser O, Jokubkiene L, Valentin L. High prevalence of defects in Cesarean section scars at transvaginal ultrasound examination. *Ultrasound Obstet Gynecol.* 2009;34:90-97.

Vikhareva Osser O, Jokubkiene L, Valentin L. Cesarean section scar defects: agreement between transvaginal sonographic findings with and without saline contrast enhancement. *Ultrasound Obstet Gynecol.* 2010;35:75-83.

C

Vikhareva Osser O, Valentin L. Clinical importance of appearance of cesarean hysterotomy scar at transvaginal ultrasonography in nonpregnant women. *Obstet Gynecol*. 2011;117:525-532.

Wang CB, Chiu WWC, Lee CY, Sun YL, Lin YH, Tseng CJ. Cesarean scar defect: correlation between Cesarean section number, defect size, clinical symptoms and uterine position. *Ultrasound Obstet Gynecol*. 2009;34:85-89.

Corpus Luteum and Hemorrhagic Cyst

Synonyms/Description
Functional cyst (corpus luteum)
No synonym for hemorrhagic cyst

Etiology
The corpus luteum (CL) is a transient structure formed as a result of ovulation, due to the mid-cycle luteinizing hormone surge from the pituitary gland. The CL is responsible for the production of progesterone, hence the term "functional cyst." It is necessary for regulating menses and for maintaining a pregnancy until it develops the ability to make its own progesterone. If a pregnancy does not occur, the CL breaks down. It can, on occasion, undergo internal hemorrhage and develop into a hemorrhagic cyst. When such a cyst continues producing progesterone, it is a hemorrhagic corpus luteum. If progesterone synthesis ceases, but the cyst persists, then it is considered a hemorrhagic cyst. Hemorrhagic cysts can enlarge up to 5 cm or more, causing pain, and may occasionally rupture, resulting in a hemoperitoneum. The pain typically resolves within a few days, whereas the cyst may take 1 to 3 months to regress. Patients with symptomatic hemorrhagic cysts typically present with acute unilateral pelvic pain and have a complex-appearing lesion on ultrasound evaluation. Often they are asymptomatic and can be an incidental finding. The nonspecific and confusing sonographic appearance of the hemorrhagic corpus luteum and hemorrhagic cyst often results in misdiagnosis and unnecessary surgery.

Ultrasound Findings
The CL is an ovarian cystic structure, typically 2 to 3 cm in size. Gray scale ultrasound characteristics include an irregular thick wall, unilocular cyst, often with internal debris or echogenic material. The most constant and specific feature of the CL is the "ring of fire" pattern of color Doppler, showing intense and abundant circumferential blood flow. The hemorrhagic CL often has a fine reticular or fishnet-like internal pattern and/or a solid area consistent with a retracting clot. Color Doppler reveals circumferential flow but no internal blood flow. The specific diagnosis is often possible sonographically, but because the CL is a mimicker of adnexal pathologies, a follow-up scan may be helpful when uncertain of the diagnosis, as discussed in clinical recommendations. A hemorrhagic cyst will have the same appearance as a hemorrhagic corpus luteum but without color flow. If internal hemorrhage occurs with cyst rupture or partial rupture, then complex fluid may be seen in the cul-de-sac or higher, or surrounding the ovary.

Differential Diagnosis
The correct diagnosis is often challenging because of variations in size, irregularity of the cyst wall, and internal solid areas (clot), all of which are nonspecific sonographic findings mimicking pathology. Knowing the menstrual cycle day is very helpful, although not always possible, in patients with irregular bleeding or menses.

In the setting of a patient presenting with pelvic pain and a tender, cystic adnexal mass, the differential diagnosis is vast and includes most commonly ectopic pregnancy, pelvic inflammatory disease (PID), adnexal torsion, and neoplasm in addition to a functional or hemorrhagic cyst. In a patient with a positive pregnancy test, the adnexal ring of an ectopic pregnancy can have a similar appearance to a CL, including the "ring of fire" Doppler pattern. Useful sonographic discriminators between these two entities are the location of the cyst and the appearance. An ectopic pregnancy typically has a more echogenic rim than a corpus luteum, and most (although not all) ectopics are extraovarian, whereas functional cysts are always in the ovary. The circumferential Doppler pattern of a corpus luteum (ring of fire) is easily distinguishable from a torsed ovary, which would typically have a paucity of flow. Doppler pattern is also a key factor in distinguishing a CL from a neoplasm. Sometimes, the retracting blood clot of a CL may have a nodular shape resembling a mural nodule. An ovarian malignant tumor will typically have blood flow visible in the internal solid area, whereas the CL only has circumferential flow with no internal Doppler signal. If the CL has undergone acute hemorrhage, the internal clot will be transiently echogenic and may be confused with a dermoid cyst. A follow-up ultrasound will be helpful because a hemorrhagic cyst will resolve, whereas the dermoid will not. Patients with PID are often clinically ill (e.g., fever, elevated white blood cell count), and the mass is typically more tubular than an ovarian cyst, often involving the fallopian tube.

Clinical Aspects and Recommendations

It is important to understand that the CL is a normal, short-lived, functional cyst found in premenopausal and pregnant women. Its function is essential, and if the corpus luteum is surgically removed in early pregnancy an abortion will ensue. Occasionally, the development of a corpus luteum may cause acute pain, even without internal hemorrhage, known as Mittelschmerz. Hemorrhage may develop within a functional cyst, resulting in acute pain, although not all hemorrhagic cysts are symptomatic. Hemorrhagic cysts will resolve over 1 to 3 months, depending on their size, as the clot is broken down and reabsorbed. If the pain and cystic mass do not resolve, the diagnosis may not be a hemorrhagic cyst (see Differential Diagnosis, earlier). It is essential to know the menstrual history, if the patient is pregnant, or if there is associated fever indicating an infection. Follow-up scans are particularly useful to track progress toward spontaneous resolution of the lesion.

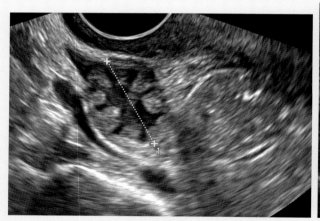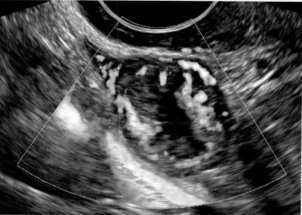

Figure C3-1 Typical corpus luteum with crenated edges, thick wall, and internal debris. The color Doppler image shows the signature intense circumferential flow of the corpus luteum.

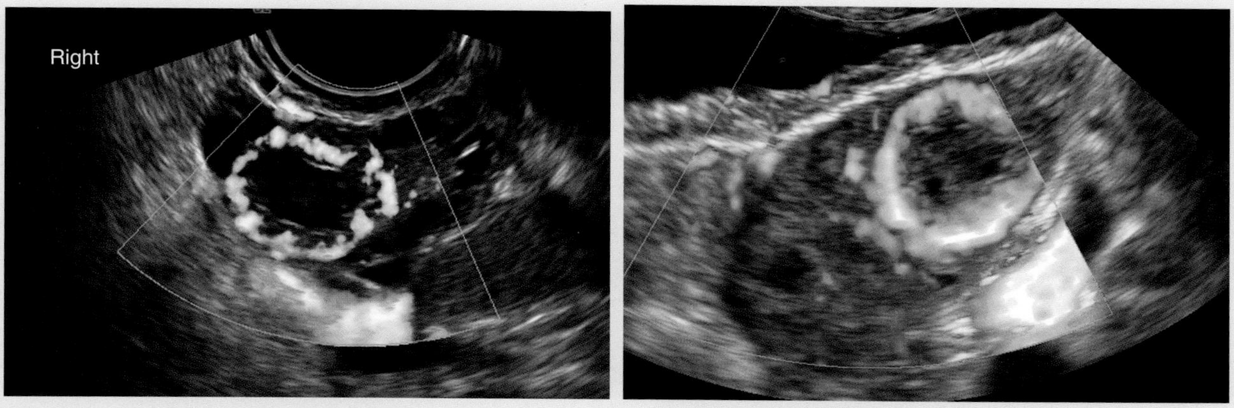

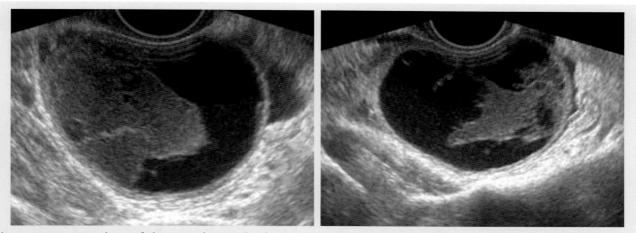

Figure C3-2   Two different patients showing the characteristic "ring of fire" flow in the corpus luteum, as seen with color Doppler.

Figure C3-3   Two views of the same hemorrhagic cyst. Note the solid areas within the cyst representing retracting clot.

C

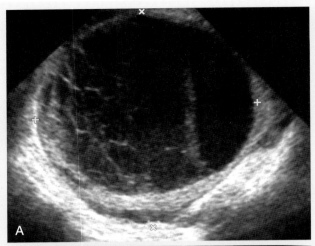

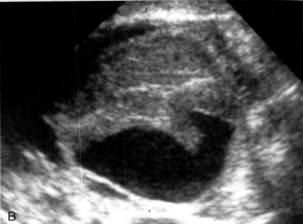

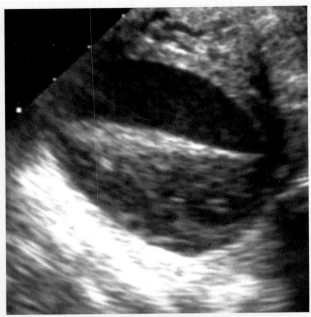

Figure C3-5   Fluid debris level in an acutely hemorrhagic cyst.

Figure C3-4   Two different cases of hemorrhagic cysts with retracting clot. **A,** The typical reticular or fishnet internal structure consistent with a retracting clot. **B,** A more solid internal structure of the cyst. Note that the solid areas are retracting toward the periphery of the cyst rather than growing into the center, as would a neoplasm. No flow was seen within the clot.

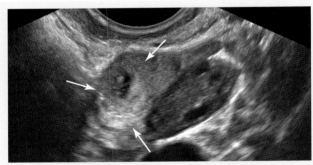

Figure C3-6   Ectopic pregnancy adjacent to a normal ovary. Note that the tubal ring is highly echogenic *(arrows)*, distinguishing it from the appearance of a corpus luteum.

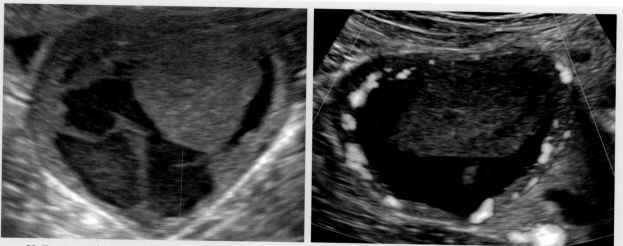

Figure C3-7   Large hemorrhagic corpus luteum with internal solid areas consistent with clot. The rounded solid areas could be confused with an ovarian neoplasm; however, the signature color Doppler "ring of fire" makes the correct diagnosis simple.

Suggested Reading

Guerriero S, Ajossa S, Melis GB. Luteal dynamics during the human menstrual cycle: new insight from imaging. *Ultrasound Obstet Gynecol.* 2005;25: 425-427.

Jain KA. Sonographic spectrum of hemorrhagic ovarian cysts. *J Ultrasound Med.* 2002;21:879-886.

Parsons AK. Imaging the human corpus luteum. *J Ultrasound Med.* 2001;20:811-819.

Stein MW, Ricci ZJ, Novak L, Roberts JH, Koenigsberg M. Sonographic comparison of the tubal ring of ectopic pregnancy with the corpus luteum. *J Ultrasound Med.* 2004;23:57-62.

Swire MN, Castro-Aragon I, Levine D. Various sonographic appearances of the hemorrhagic corpus luteum cyst. *Ultrasound Q.* 2004;20:45-58.

Cyst, Clear

Synonyms/Description
Simple cyst
Clear ovarian cyst

Etiology
A simple ovarian cyst is a clear, thin-walled, unilocular cyst.

Premenopausal
Simple cysts up to 3 cm in maximal diameter are considered normal physiologic follicles in cycling women, and thus should not be reported as a cyst, particularly when the patient is midcycle. If a clear simple cyst does not resolve, it may be extraovarian, specifically paraovarian or paratubal. A persistent thin-walled and unilocular cyst may also represent a serous cystadenoma.

Postmenopausal
Small simple cysts up to 1 cm may be seen in up to 21% of postmenopausal women, and these are not considered clinically significant, even though the patient is no longer cycling. These less than 1 cm cysts typically should not be reported on an ultrasound examination and do not require follow-up.

In a study by Greenlee and colleagues, 2217 (14.1%) out of 15,735 women screened sonographically had one or more simple cysts on ultrasound examination. Among women without a cyst on the first screen, 8.3% had a new simple cyst 1 year later. There was no statistical difference in rate of subsequent ovarian cancer when those with simple cysts were compared with those without a cyst.

Ultrasound Findings
A simple and clear ovarian cyst is a thin, smooth-walled structure containing fluid with no internal echoes or solid areas. The cyst is usually round but can be oval, especially as it regresses and changes shape.

Any cyst that has a thick wall or any solid component is in a different category and discussed in other sections (refer to the differential diagnosis list for a complex cyst).

It is very important to scrutinize the sonographic appearance of cysts for any solid components or areas of wall thickening. A study by Valentin reports that 11 (0.96%) out of 1148 masses classified as unilocular cysts on ultrasound were malignant. However, postoperatively, 7 of the 11 malignancies thought to be unilocular cysts on ultrasound had gross papillary projections on the surgical specimen. Therefore accurate classification of a cyst as clear and unilocular is crucial on ultrasound examinations. Color Doppler may be useful to interrogate the walls of a cyst to better demonstrate any wall irregularity.

Differential Diagnosis
In a premenopausal patient, a simple cyst is most likely follicular and thus functional. If the patient is postmenopausal or the cyst does not regress in 3 months, the differential diagnosis includes cystadenoma, paratubal or paraovarian cyst, hydrosalpinx, or peritoneal inclusion cyst. Occasionally, serous cystadenomas can be unilocular and thin walled, although some may have a worrisome component such as a focally thick wall or septations. Paratubal or paraovarian cysts may mimic a follicle but can be distinguished sonographically by their location off the edge, or distant, from the ovary. Hydrosalpinges are rarely clear and thin walled, and are usually tubular with incomplete septations. Peritoneal inclusion cysts develop as a result of fluid being trapped within peritoneal adhesions. They typically have thin walls, an odd shape and may have multiple thin septations—all clues to the correct diagnosis.

Clinical Aspects and Recommendations
In general, simple clear cysts do not convey an increased risk of ovarian cancer, even in

postmenopausal patients. With benign epithelial ovarian lesions there is no indication that malignant transformation occurs; for example, cystadenomas do not become cystadenocarcinomas. Current recommendations for management of simple cysts are the result of a collaborative consensus panel hosted by the Society of Radiologists in Ultrasound. The following recommendations pertain only to thin smooth-walled, completely clear, unilocular cysts.

In Premenopausal Women

Cysts less than 3 cm are considered normal and need not be followed. Cysts measuring 3 to 5 cm should be reported with a statement that they are almost certainly benign and may not need follow-up. Cysts between 5 and 7 cm are almost certainly benign but should be followed yearly with ultrasound. Cysts larger than 7 cm may be difficult to evaluate completely sonographically and might warrant further imaging.

In Postmenopausal Women

Cysts less than 1 cm are clinically inconsequential and may not be reported.

Cysts between 1 and 7 cm should be reported with a statement that they are almost certainly

benign sonographically and yearly follow-up is recommended.

Cysts larger than 7 cm may be difficult to assess fully with ultrasound; thus surgical evaluation or alternative imaging should be considered.

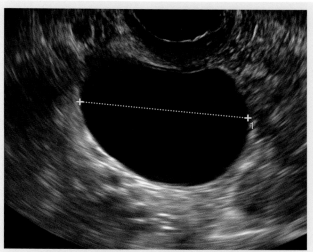

Figure C4-2   Five-centimeter unilocular simple cyst showing the characteristic thin smooth walls and anechoic internal structure.

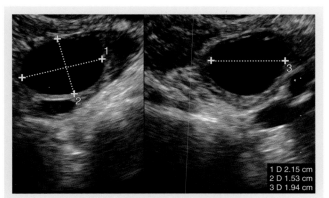

Figure C4-1   Two views of a thin-walled unilocular cyst. This is a dominant follicle and is entirely normal. Such a cyst should not be mentioned in the ultrasound report because it is a normal finding.

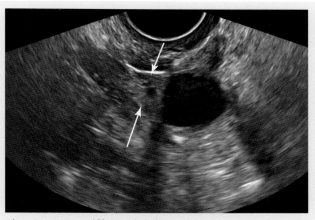

Figure C4-3   Differential diagnosis—paraovarian cyst (see Paratubal or Paraovarian Cysts). Note that the unilocular cyst is located adjacent to the ovary *(arrows)*.

C

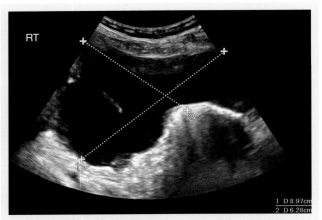

Figure C4-4 Differential diagnosis of large perito-neal inclusion cyst (see the section on complex cysts). This cyst is neither totally anechoic nor unilocular. It seems to take on the shape of the peritoneal space, a characteristic that is typical of a peritoneal inclusion cyst secondary to adhesions after pelvic surgery.

Suggested Reading

Greenlee RT, Kessel B, Williams CR, Riley TL, Ragard LR, Hartge P, Buys SS, Partridge EE, Reding DJ. Prevalence, incidence, and natural history of simple ovarian cysts among women >55 years old in a large cancer screening trial. *Am J Obstet Gynecol.* 2010;202:373.e1-9.

Levine D, Brown DL, Andreotti RF, Benacerraf B, Benson CB, Brewster WR, Coleman B, DePriest P, Doubilet PM, Goldstein SR, Hamper UM, Hecht JL, Horrow M, Hur HC, Marnach M, Patel MD, Platt LD, Puscheck E, Smith-Bindman R. Society of Radiologists in Ultrasound. Management of asymptomatic ovarian and other adnexal cysts imaged at US Society of Radiologists in Ultrasound consensus conference statement. *Ultrasound Q.* 2010;26:121-131.

Valentin L, Ameye L, Franchi D, Guerriero S, Jurkovic D, Savelli L, Fischerova D, Lissoni A, Van Holsbeke C, Fruscio R, Van Huffel S, Testa A, Timmerman D. Risk of malignancy in unilocular cysts: a study of 1148 adnexal masses classified as unilocular cysts at transvaginal ultrasound and review of the literature. *Ultrasound Obstet Gynecol.* 2013;41:80-89.

Cystadenofibroma

Synonyms/Description
Benign ovarian tumor that arises from surface epithelium and underlying cortical connective tissue of the ovary.

Etiology
These are rare benign ovarian tumors representing less than 2% of benign ovarian neoplasms. Originally thought to be fibrous variants of cystadenomas (the most common benign epithelial ovarian neoplasms), these tumors actually originate from the surface epithelium as well as the underlying cortical connective tissue of the ovary.

Ultrasound Findings
Cystadenofibromas are often complex in their sonographic appearance. They are at least partly if not predominantly cystic and may contain septations, solid areas, and nodularity. The most common appearance (69% in a series of 58 cases) is a unilocular cyst with papillations that project into the lumen but do not demonstrate blood flow using color Doppler. The appearance, however, can be quite variable, and can mimic the appearance of a malignancy, with thick septations and blood flow in the solid areas. Occasionally, ovarian cystadenofibromas may be borderline tumors (5 in a series of 47 tumors).

Differential Diagnosis
In some patients, the tumor has an appearance indistinguishable from a malignancy, with solid areas and septations containing color flow on Doppler evaluation; these are usually removed. The majority of cystadenofibromas are unilocular with solid areas devoid of blood flow. The main differential diagnosis includes an endometrioma or a cystadenoma (mucinous or serous).

Clinical Aspects and Recommendations
Like most adnexal masses, such tumors are usually discovered at the time of bimanual examination or incidentally during pelvic imaging. Less commonly they can be associated with pelvic pain, which may be a result of enlargement of the mass. Unlike fibroadenomas, which are primarily solid tumors, the epithelial portion of cystadenofibromas always has a cystic component. The presence of papillary projections (solid mural nodules) emanating from the cyst wall may raise concerns about potential malignancy. However, emerging clinical evidence suggests that when cystadenofibromas present as a unilocular cystic structure with a small avascular mural nodule, conservative management may be a more appropriate approach.

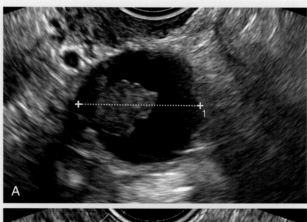

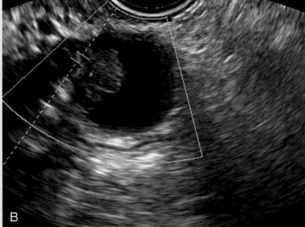

Figure C5-1 **A,** Typical appearance of a cystadenofibroma: a unilocular cyst with a solid nodule. **B,** The nodule contains a paucity of blood flow by color Doppler.

C

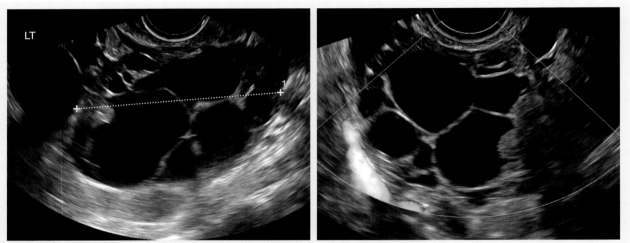

Figure C5-2   Atypical appearance of a cystadenofibroma appearing as a multiseptate cystic mass with solid components. A paucity of blood flow is demonstrated in the solid areas, although scant blood flow is present in the septae.

Suggested Reading

Tang YZ, Liyanage S, Narayanan P, Sahdev A, Sohaib A, Singh N, Rockall A. The MRI features of histologically proven ovarian cystadenofibromas-an assessment of the morphological and enhancement patterns. *Eur Radiol.* 2013;23:48-56.

Washish A, Elsayes K. Ovarian cystadenofibroma: a masquerader of malignancy. *Indian J Radiol Imag.* 2010;20:297-299.

Dermoid Cyst

Synonyms/Description
Mature cystic teratoma

Etiology
This is a benign germ cell tumor containing ectoderm, mesoderm, and endoderm, thought to arise from a single germ cell. Components may include hair, teeth, fat, and bone. These tumors represent 25% of all ovarian neoplasms and 60% of all benign ovarian tumors. They are bilateral and or recurrent in 10% of cases. These lesions are benign and typically occur in teenagers and young adults, although approximately 1% may be immature teratomas with malignant components mixed with mature elements.

Ultrasound Findings
The classic sonographic appearance of a dermoid is an echogenic mass with intense acoustic shadowing obscuring the back wall. A finding coined "tip of the iceberg" refers to this characteristic, which can make obtaining accurate measurements of the mass difficult. The intensely echogenic components of dermoid cysts represent varying combinations of fat, sebaceous material, hair, teeth, and bone. There are often a multitude of thin echogenic lines emanating from the echogenic center representing strands of hair within the mass. The so-called "Rokitansky nodule" is a very echogenic, discrete, rounded protuberance characteristic of a dermoid. There is typically no demonstrable blood flow within these lesions.

Less commonly, dermoids can be predominantly cystic with only a small echogenic nodule that is easy to miss and that indicates the correct diagnosis. There can be septations and low-level echoes, which may be confused as findings consistent with an endometrioma. Occasionally, dermoids can be made up of a multitude of small round balls within a mass, like a cluster of billiard balls. This is rare but when visualized is a characteristic appearance of a dermoid cyst.

Differential Diagnosis
The diagnosis of a dermoid is very specific when the appearance is characteristic. When the appearance is not typical, dermoids can be mistaken for endometriomas, fibromas, and struma ovarii. The absence of color flow on Doppler examination is a very important and helpful feature of dermoids. If a dermoid is suspected but color flow is observed in the solid areas, other etiologies must be considered. The sonographic appearance of the rarer malignant teratoma is similar to the mature lesions except for the Doppler pattern of blood flow. This is rarely seen in the benign lesions but common in malignancies. The short growth interval of the lesion may also suggest a malignancy.

Clinical Aspects and Recommendations
Most dermoid cysts are asymptomatic. If symptoms are present, it often depends on the size of the mass. Such ovarian pathology is not usually associated with adhesion formation, and adnexal torsion can occur, especially if the cyst is large. They rarely rupture, but when they do, spillage of sebaceous material into the abdominal cavity may cause chemical peritonitis and development of dense intra-abdominal adhesions. This rare complication can present with acute symptoms, but the most common cause of acute pelvic pain in the presence of a dermoid is torsion.

Malignant transformation, although extremely rare (quoted to be 0.2% to 2% in such benign teratomas), can occur. This is unlike epithelial ovarian neoplasms, in which benign growths do not transform into malignant ones.

Ovarian cystectomy is the treatment of choice in reproductive-age women when intervention is indicated. This allows for a definitive diagnosis, preservation of ovarian tissue, and decreased risk of torsion or rupture. For those women who have completed their child bearing, salpingo-oophorectomy is an acceptable treatment option. There is a 10% to 20% incidence of bilaterality, and a thorough ultrasound examination of the nonaffected ovary preoperatively should be carried out rather than the historical approach of bivalving that ovary.

D

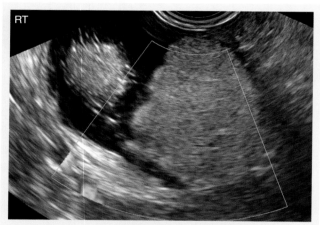

Figure D1-1 Dermoid. Large mass with typical round echogenic foci and thin linear strands emanating from the center. Note the lack of color flow in the solid portions.

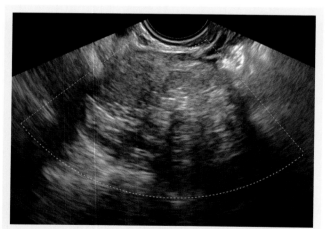

Figure D1-2 Dermoid. Typical heterogeneous echogenic mass with shadowing obscuring posterior wall.

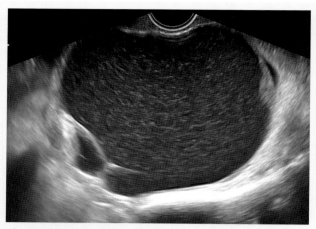

Figure D1-3 Predominantly cystic dermoid mimicking an endometrioma. The small echogenic nodule along the right side of the mass is a clue to the correct diagnosis.

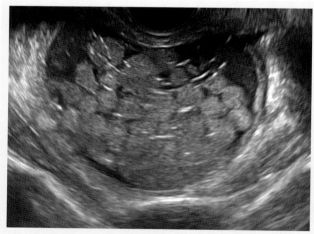

Figure D1-4 Unusual but characteristic appearance of a dermoid, containing a cluster of small solid spheres representing small balls of fat.

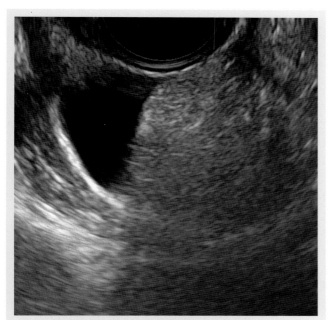

Figure D1-5 Cystic mass with typical echogenic rounded component with intense shadowing. This typical dermoid was located in the cul-de-sac unrelated to either ovary. At surgery it proved to be a parasitic dermoid of the rectovaginal septum.

Suggested Reading

Outwater EK, Siegelman ES, Hunt JL. Ovarian teratomas: tumor types and imaging characteristics. *Radiographics.* 2001;21:475-490.

Sokalska A, Timmerman D, Testa AC, Van Holsbeke C, Lissoni AA, Leone FP, Jurkovic D, Valentin L. Diagnostic accuracy of transvaginal ultrasound examination for assigning a specific diagnosis to adnexal masses. *Ultrasound Obstet Gynecol.* 2009;34: 462-470.

Ushakov FB, Meirow D, Prus D, Libson E, BenShushan A, Rojansky N. Parasitic ovarian dermoid tumor of the omentum. A review of the literature and report of two new cases. *Eur J Obstet Gynecol Reprod Biol.* 1998;81:77-82. Review.

Dysgerminoma

Synonyms/Description

Malignant germ cell tumor diagnosed predominantly in young adults ages 20 to 30. The most common benign germ cell tumor is the mature teratoma, commonly called a dermoid cyst (see Dermoid Cyst).

Etiology

Primitive germ cell tumors include the dysgerminoma, immature teratoma, endodermal sinus/yolk sac tumor, embryonal carcinoma, and nongestational choriocarcinoma.

Ovarian dysgerminomas arise from primordial germ cells and represent 1% to 2% of ovarian malignancies and 30% of all malignant germ cell tumors. Dysgerminoma is a rare tumor similar in histology to the male testicular seminoma and can arise bilaterally in 15% of affected patients. Serum human chorionic gonadotropin (hCG) is occasionally elevated.

Ultrasound Findings

Findings involve a solid, mostly isoechoic, but heterogeneous mass with apparent lobulations. The lobulations are caused by inhomogeneous internal echogenicity giving the sonographic appearance of different compartments in this solid tumor. Blood flow is moderate to abundant in most lesions, indicating a high risk of malignancy.

Differential Diagnosis

The solid appearance of this tumor makes the differential diagnosis extensive. Struma ovarii (ectopic thyroid tissue, monodermal teratoma) can have a similar appearance although less vascular. Other solid ovarian malignancies should be considered, including metastatic disease to the ovary, lymphoma, and predominantly solid cystadenocarcinomas (although the common cystic portions of these cystadenocarcinomas are not usually seen in dysgerminomas). The extensive blood flow makes the fibroma and mature dermoid unlikely.

Clinical Aspects and Recommendations

Dysgerminomas may present either as palpable adnexal masses or as incidental findings on an imaging study. Occasionally, these tumors display unusually rapid growth, and patients may present with abdominal enlargement and pain caused by rupture with hemoperitoneum or torsion. If the tumor is hormonally active, menstrual abnormalities may occur. These tumors can produce placental alkaline phosphatase and LDH. Thus, in patients with a solid-appearing adnexal mass, assessment of such tumor markers may be helpful. An occasional patient may produce hCG but virtually never produces alpha fetoprotein (AFP). Studies indicate that approximately 75% of women with dysgerminomas present with stage I disease. There is bilateral involvement in approximately 10% to 15% of cases. Because the ultrasound findings are nonspecific, treatment is surgical exploration and resection in virtually all cases. These patients are often young and have not completed their child bearing; therefore, unilateral salpingo-oophorectomy is appropriate and is curative in most cases.

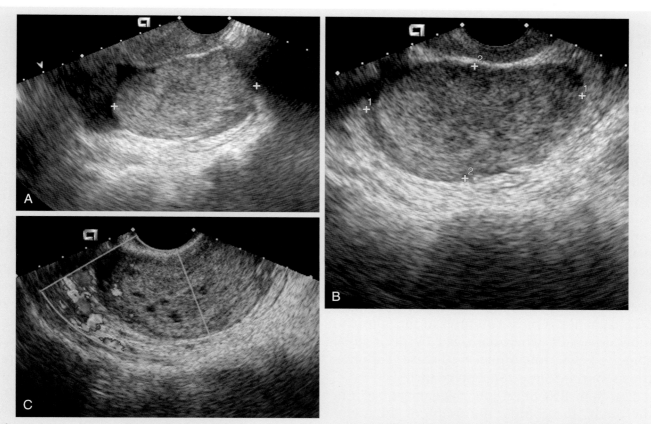

Figure D2-1   Dysgerminoma (two patients). **A and B,** Solid rounded lobular ovarian mass with no visible cystic component. **C,** Color flow Doppler of the mass shows blood flow pattern in a different patient with dysgerminoma.

Suggested Reading

Gordon A, Lipton D, Woodruff JD. Dysgerminoma: a review of 158 cases from the Emil Novak Ovarian Tumor Registry. *Obstet Gynecol.* 1981;58:497-504.

Guerriero S, Testa AC, Timmerman D, Van Holsbeke C, Ajossa S, Fischerova D, Franchi D, Leone FP, Domali E, Alcazar JL, Parodo G, Mascilini F, Virgilio B, Demidov VN, Lipatenkova J, Valentin L. Imaging of gynecological disease (6): clinical and ultrasound characteristics of ovarian dysgerminoma. *Ultrasound Obstet Gynecol.* 2011;37:596-602.

Kim SH, Kang SB. Ovarian dysgerminoma: color Doppler ultrasonographic findings and comparison with CT and MR imaging findings. *J Ultrasound Med.* 1995;14:843-848.

Vicus D, Beiner ME, Klachook S, Le LW, Laframboise S, Mackay H. Pure dysgerminoma of the ovary 35 years on: a single institutional experience. *Gynecol Oncol.* 2010;117:23-26.

Ectopic Pregnancy

Synonyms/Description
Tubal, cornual, cervical, ovarian, or abdominal pregnancy/ectopic

Etiology
An ectopic pregnancy is a pregnancy that occurs as a result of implantation of a fertilized ovum outside the endometrial cavity. Ectopic pregnancy occurs in approximately 1.5% to 2.0% of gestations and can be life threatening, accounting for 6% of all maternal deaths because of late presentation or unrecognized symptoms. Ectopic pregnancy is most common in the fallopian tube, especially when damaged by prior tubal surgery, pelvic inflammatory disease, endometriosis, or previous ectopic pregnancies.

Less than 10% of ectopic pregnancies occur in the cervix, the cornua, the ovary, or the abdomen. These are more difficult to diagnose and treat, thus resulting in higher morbidity than tubal pregnancies. More recently, implantation in Cesarean section scars has been described with increasing frequency.

Ultrasound Findings
Transvaginal ultrasonography has 73% to 93% sensitivity for diagnosing ectopic pregnancy, depending on sonographer expertise and gestational age. On rare occasions, there is a gestational sac with a live embryo in the adnexa and the sonographic diagnosis of an ectopic pregnancy can be definitive. In 8% to 31% of women suspected of having an ectopic pregnancy, the initial ultrasound does not show the whereabouts of the pregnancy (pregnancy of unknown location [PUL]).

An empty-appearing uterus may indicate an intrauterine pregnancy too early to see (less than 5 weeks), a failed pregnancy too small or already passed, or an ectopic pregnancy. Technical factors such as fibroids, adenomyosis, morbid obesity, or an axial uterus may make imaging more difficult. Approximately 7% to 20% of women presenting with a PUL are ultimately diagnosed with ectopic pregnancy.

When there is no visible intrauterine pregnancy, it is important to determine the level of human chorionic gonadotropin (hCG). Serial hCG levels are necessary when evaluating pregnancies of unknown location to observe the trend. In a normal early pregnancy, hCG levels will rise by at least 53%, but typically greater than or equal to 100% (99% confidence interval) every 48 hours. Most ectopic pregnancies are associated with a low and abnormally slow rising hCG level. The reported "discriminatory hCG value" at which an intrauterine pregnancy must be identified sonographically has varied in the literature between 1000 and 3000 mIU/mm. It is probable that a patient with an empty uterus and an hCG level of greater than 3000 mIU/mm has an ectopic pregnancy unless she has had a recent complete spontaneous abortion between the time of the hCG and the sonogram.

In the absence of an intrauterine pregnancy, the most common sonographic signs of a tubal pregnancy include an adnexal mass (heterogeneous cystic and/or solid), a tubal ring (small round cyst with echogenic rim), a tubular mass consistent with a hematosalpinx, and echogenic free fluid in the cul-de-sac consistent with blood. Color Doppler often shows circumferential flow around a tubal ring, similar to a corpus luteum, but there is typically no flow inside a hematosalpinx. It is helpful to distinguish the ovary as separate from the ectopic pregnancy mass so as not to misdiagnose the mass as ovarian in origin. Pushing the mass gently past the ovary can demonstrate that they are separate.

Cornual ectopic pregnancies account for 1% to 6% of ectopic pregnancies and can be diagnosed if the gestational sac is located clearly outside of the endometrial cavity but surrounded by a thin rim of myometrium. If there is myometrium between the gestational sac and the endometrial cavity, then the pregnancy is cornual.

Cervical ectopic pregnancies account for less than 1% of ectopics and are diagnosed when the gestational sac is clearly seen within the cervix. A sac can slide through the cervix during a spontaneous pregnancy loss; therefore if this is suspected, a follow-up scan in 24 hours may be necessary to confirm a cervical pregnancy. Blood flow is typically present around the sac of a pregnancy implanted in the cervix as opposed to an ongoing pregnancy loss in which circumferential blood flow is absent.

Cesarean section scar pregnancies account for up to 6% of ectopic gestations in women with prior Cesarean sections. The gestational sac is typically located low and anterior, just cephalad to the internal os, obliterating the site of the C-section scar. The sac deforms the anterior lower uterine segment, causing an anterior bulge, with very little myometrium, if any, stretched around the outer surface of the sac, bringing it adjacent to the bladder.

Although the presence of an intrauterine pregnancy is good evidence against the presence of an ectopic pregnancy, the presence of a heterotopic pregnancy (co-existing intrauterine and extrauterine pregnancies) is possible, and is more common with the use of assisted reproduction. The sonographic signs of ectopic pregnancy should be sought even if an intrauterine pregnancy is present.

Differential Diagnosis
The diagnosis of ectopic pregnancy depends entirely on the presence of a positive pregnancy test, which is an essential finding before a differential diagnosis is attempted.

An ectopic pregnancy can masquerade as a hydrosalpinx, pelvic inflammatory disease, endometriosis, appendicitis, ovarian tumor, degenerating pedunculated fibroid, and so on. In the setting of a positive pregnancy test and no visible intrauterine pregnancy, an adnexal lesion should raise suspicion for an ectopic pregnancy. A cervical pregnancy may be confused with an ongoing spontaneous abortion. Doppler is useful to determine whether the sac is attached in the cervix or just passing through. A cornual pregnancy may mimic a degenerating fibroid, but the clinical history and pregnancy test should contribute to the correct diagnosis.

Clinical Aspects and Recommendations
Many tubal ectopic pregnancies can be treated with methotrexate. Before injecting such an agent to terminate the pregnancy in a patient with PUL, there must be no possibility that the pregnancy could still be intrauterine. Even if the uterus is empty on the initial ultrasound, serial hCGs and follow-up ultrasounds are often needed in a stable patient to be certain that an early intrauterine pregnancy is not overlooked. Methotrexate will irrevocably destroy trophoblastic tissue and potentially damage a desired intrauterine pregnancy. Cervical and cornual pregnancies are typically injected with methotrexate or potassium chloride directly into the sac or embryo to provide local and direct treatment. Sometimes follow-up methotrexate injections are necessary. Ultimately, patients may need laparoscopy if medical treatment fails. Laparoscopy is usually necessary with large tubal pregnancies or those in which cardiac activity is present. The treatment for C-section scar ectopics depends on multiple factors and includes medical and surgical approaches.

E

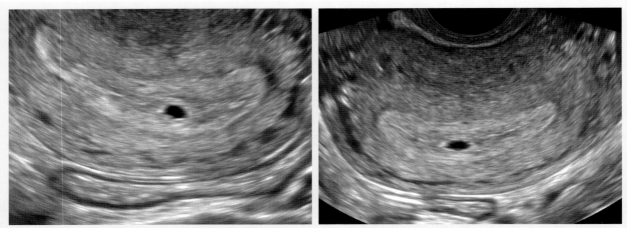

Figure E1-1   Intrauterine pregnancy. Longitudinal and transverse views of the uterus showing a small 5-week-size gestational sac. The rounded sac with echogenic rim within the decidua is the earliest visible indication of an intrauterine pregnancy.

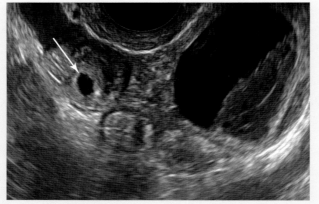

Figure E1-2   Tubal ectopic pregnancy. View of the right adnexa showing a hemorrhagic cyst within the ovary, adjacent to which is a small ectopic pregnancy *(arrow)*. Note the intense echogenic rim of the ectopic sac, compared with the echolucent border of the hemorrhagic corpus luteum.

E

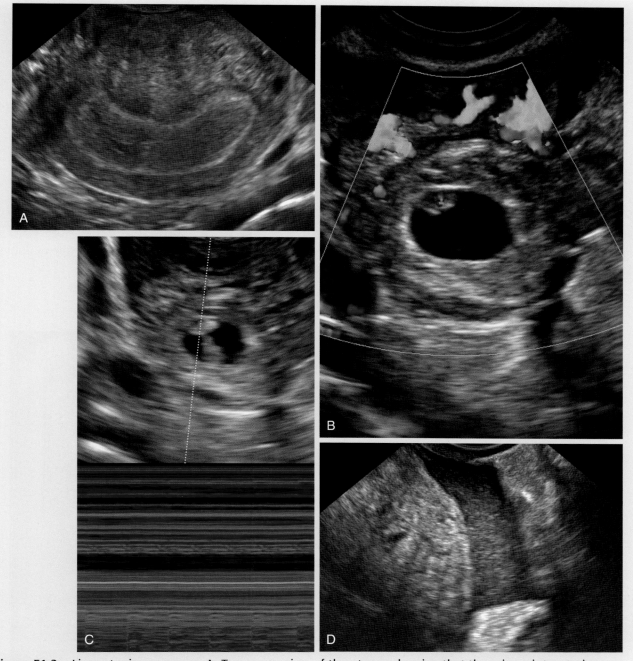

Figure E1-3   Live ectopic pregnancy. **A,** Transverse view of the uterus, showing that there is no intrauterine pregnancy. **B and C,** A live ectopic pregnancy with a gestational sac and an embryo in the adnexa. The embryo has a heartbeat seen with Doppler and m-mode. **D,** A moderate amount of echogenic free fluid in the cul-de-sac of the same patient, indicating leakage of blood from the ectopic pregnancy.

E

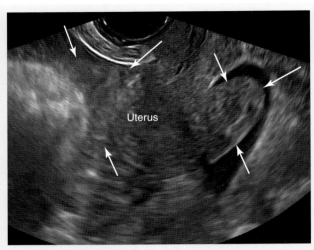

Figure E1-4   Longitudinal view of an empty uterus in a patient with a ruptured ectopic pregnancy. Note multiple blood clots *(arrows)*, both in front of and behind the uterus.

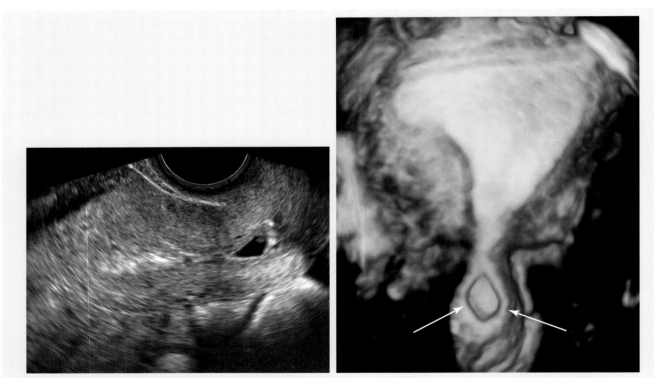

Figure E1-5   Cervical pregnancy. Longitudinal view and 3-D rendering of a 5-week cervical pregnancy. Note the presence of the gestational sac within the cervix (*arrows* on 3-D view).

E

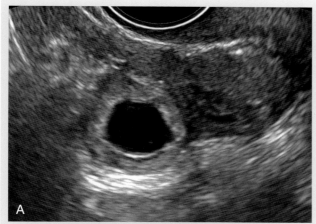

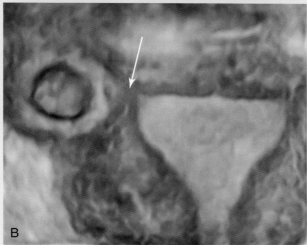

Figure E1-6 Cornual pregnancy. **A,** The gestational sac with its echogenic rim, located adjacent to the fundus of the uterus. **B,** A 3-D rendered image showing the proximity of the cornual ectopic sac to the endometrial cavity. The arrow demonstrates a thin tongue of myometrium separating the sac and the edge of the cavity.

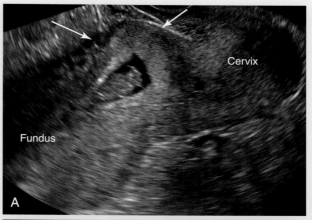

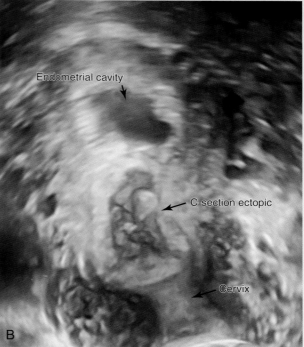

Figure E1-7 C-section scar ectopic pregnancy. **A,** A longitudinal view of a uterus with a C-section scar ectopic pregnancy located in the anterior lower uterine segment. Note the anterior bulge made by the invading trophoblast *(arrows)*. There is no visible myometrium seen around the outside of the sac. **B,** The coronal view of the uterus using 3-D rendering. Note the location of the pregnancy in the lower uterine segment.

E

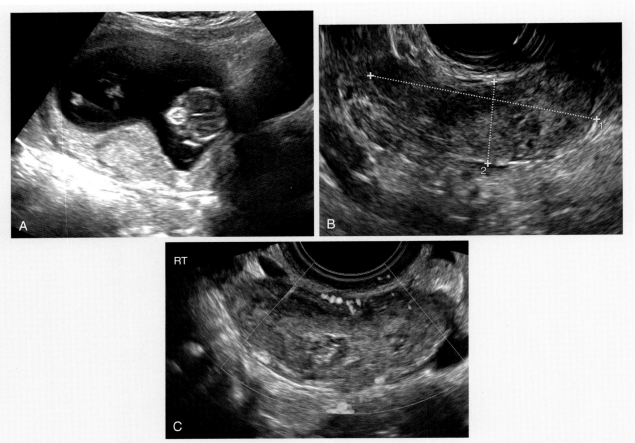

Figure E1-8   Heterotopic pregnancy at 12 weeks. **A,** The normal intrauterine pregnancy at 12 weeks. **B and C,** A tubular solid mass in the right adnexa of the same patient. Note that there is only peripheral vascularity and no blood flow in the center of the mass. This was an ectopic pregnancy with a hematosalpinx in the setting of a co-existing intrauterine pregnancy.

Suggested Reading

Barnhart KT. Ectopic pregnancy. *N Engl J Med.* 2009; 361:379-387.

Kamaya A, Shin L, Chen B, Desser TS. Emergency gynecologic imaging. *Semin Ultrasound CT MRI.* 2008;29:353-368.

Kirk E, Bourne T. Diagnosis of ectopic pregnancy with ultrasound. *Best Pract Res Clin Obstet Gynaecol.* 2009;23:501-508.

Lin EP, Bhatt S, Dogra VS. Diagnostic clues to ectopic pregnancy. *RadioGraphics.* 2008;28:1661-1671.

Osborn DA, Williams TR, Craig BM. Cesarean scar pregnancy: sonographic and magnetic resonance imaging findings, complications, and treatment. *J Ultrasound Med.* 2012;31:1449-1456.

Endometrial Carcinoma

Synonyms/Description
Uterine cancer

Etiology
Endometrial cancer is the most common cancer of the female genital tract. The overall 5-year survival rate is 85%, 75%, 45%, and 25% for stages I through IV, respectively.

Risk factors for endometrial cancer include obesity, diabetes, nulliparity, estrogen-producing ovarian tumors, polycystic ovarian syndrome, advanced age, unopposed estrogen therapy, tamoxifen, and a family history of nonpolypoid colorectal cancer.

The prognosis depends on the tumor type and stage. Type 1 endometrial cancer or endometrioid carcinoma accounts for 80% of uterine carcinomas and is associated with increased and unopposed estrogen exposure. It typically arises from a background of endometrial hyperplasia and is frequently low-grade and slow-growing.

Type 2 tumors are not estrogen driven and are generally far more aggressive than type 1. They often occur in the setting of atrophic endometrium and include serous, clear cell, and other cell types. These tumors tend to invade the myometrium earlier and spread rapidly.

Ultrasound Findings
The gray-scale sonographic appearance of endometrial cancer depends on the stage of disease. If the tumor is confined to the endometrium and small, the scan may reveal a thickened, heterogeneous endometrium or even a normal-appearing endometrium if the tumor is very small. In postmenopausal patients who are bleeding, an endometrial thickness greater than 4 mm (some use greater than or equal to 5 mm) is considered abnormal and requires further evaluation. Early-stage tumors are typically hyperechoic and may have some but limited color flow within the endometrium. If the endometrium appears abnormal or ill defined, a sonohysterogram can be performed to outline the endometrium and determine whether there is a focal or diffuse process.

More advanced tumors often have a texture of mixed echogenicity and abundant vascularity evident on color Doppler. The tumor vessels are typically multiple, disorganized, and entering from multiple foci. As the tumor continues to grow, the borders become increasingly irregular and ill-defined, invading the myometrium, with loss of definition of the endometrial-myometrial junction. There can be cystic spaces within the characteristically solid tumor and, sometimes, fluid in the endometrial cavity outlining the mass. As the endometrial tumor invades further into the myometrium, the uterus enlarges and becomes blotchy in texture. With extensive myometrial invasion, the residual mantle of myometrium may be very thin. Some tumors seem to be entirely in the myometrium rather than the endometrium (see Figure E2-3).

Endometrial cancer can arise not only in the uterine fundus (most common), but also in the lower uterine segment, at the cervical junction, distorting the shape of the lower segment (see Figure E2-5).

Differential Diagnosis
When the endometrial abnormality is confined to the endometrium and appears typically echogenic, the differential diagnosis includes polyps and endometrial hyperplasia. A sonohysterogram is very helpful as the initial workup for a thickened or ill-defined endometrium in a patient with abnormal or postmenopausal bleeding. The age, history, and hormonal status of the patient are important factors to consider, but tissue sampling is necessary when malignancy is being considered. The differential diagnosis for a uterine mass with irregular cystic areas and excessive vascularity includes sarcoma and fibroids (see Uterine Sarcoma and also Fibroids). Because fibroids are far more common than uterine cancers, a uterine

mass may be mistaken for an atypical fibroid at first scan. If a fibroid is unusual in appearance, it is important to rescan the patient in a relatively short time interval to evaluate growth of the lesion. Adenomyosis can give the myometrium a focal blotchy appearance, although the vascularity should differentiate adenomyosis from a cancer.

Clinical Aspects and Recommendations

Endometrial cancer is typically treated with total abdominal hysterectomy, bilateral salpingo-oophorectomy, and staging, which includes lymph node sampling. Further therapy depends on the stage and type of tumor; it may involve gynecologic, radiation, and medical oncologists.

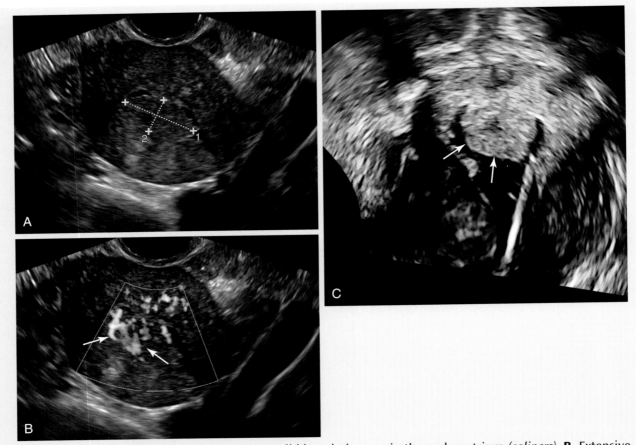

Figure E2-1   Polypoid endometrial cancer. **A,** A solid isoechoic mass in the endometrium *(calipers).* **B,** Extensive color flow displaying multiple, irregular vessels in the mass *(arrows).* **C,** A 3-D coronal rendering of the uterus after saline had been introduced into the cavity. Note the tumor *(arrows)* at the fundus of the uterus, outlined by fluid.

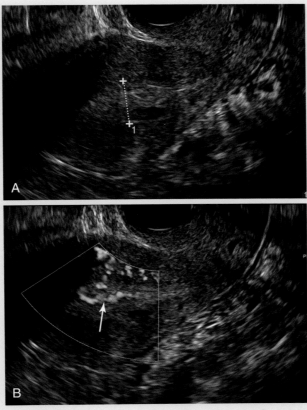

Figure E2-2   A, Longitudinal view of the uterus in a patient with adenocarcinoma of the endometrium. Note the thick and heterogeneous endometrium with ill-defined borders on the gray scale image. **B,** The color flow image shows abundant vascularity *(arrow)* in the endometrium.

E

E

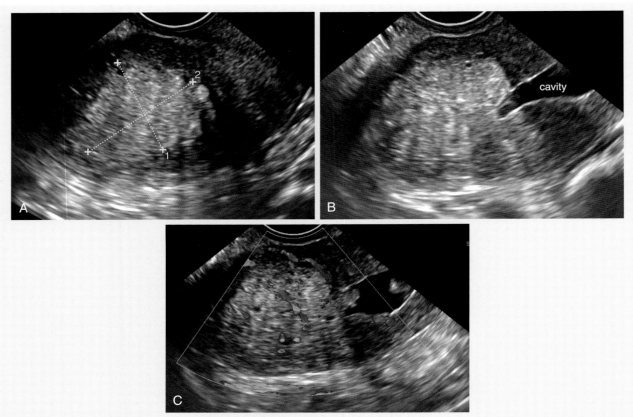

Figure E2-3   A and B, Large echogenic endometrial cancer *(calipers)* invading the myometrium with only a small component in the endometrial cavity. **C,** The color flow image shows the abundant vascularity in this aggressive tumor.

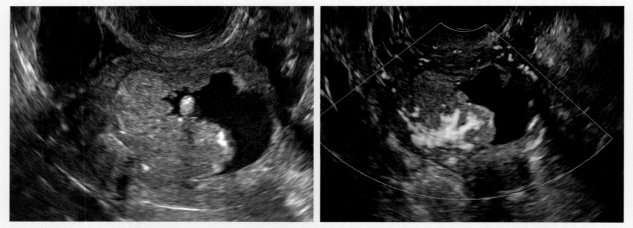

Figure E2-4   Large endometrial cancer located within the endometrial cavity and involving approximately 50% of the circumference of the endometrium. This mass is protruding into the cavity and outlined by endometrial fluid. Note the intense vascularity evident on the color flow image.

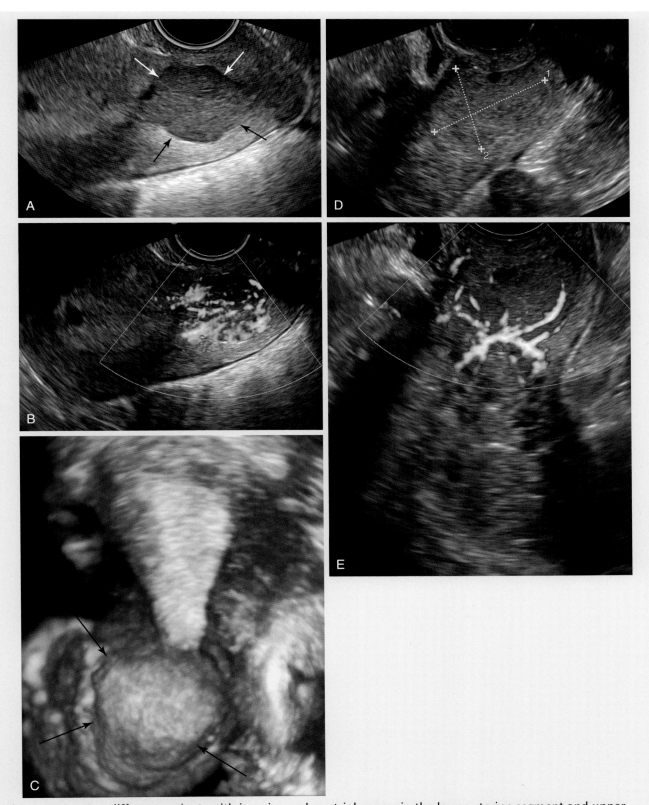

Figure E2-5 Two different patients with invasive endometrial cancer in the lower uterine segment and upper cervix. **A and B,** A solid, homogeneous mass *(arrows)* that is very vascular and located in the lower uterine segment and involving the upper portion of the cervix. **C,** The 3-D coronal view of the same mass showing its location in the lower portion of the uterus as well as its irregular contour *(arrows).* **D and E,** A different patient with a similar tumor *(calipers)* in the lower uterus/cervix. Note the disorganized abundant vascularity to the mass.

E

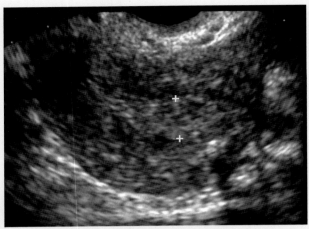

Figure E2-6 Endometrium of a 75-year-old asymptomatic woman who was on unopposed estrogen for more than 10 years. Despite the absence of bleeding, this endometrium of 8 mm was considered heterogeneous and abnormal, prompting sampling. Stage Ib endometrial carcinoma was diagnosed, invading one third of the way through the myometrium (invasion not detectable sonographically).

Videos
Video 1 on endometrial carcinoma is available online.

Suggested Reading

Amant F, Moerman P, Neven P, Timmerman D, Van Limbergen E, Vergote I. Endometrial cancer. *Lancet.* 2005;366:491-505.

Epstein E, Van Holsbeke C, Mascilini F, Måsbäck A, Kannisto P, Ameye L, Fischerova D, Zannoni G, Vellone V, Timmerman D, Testa AC. Gray-scale and color Doppler ultrasound characteristics of endometrial cancer in relation to stage, grade and tumor size. *Ultrasound Obstet Gynecol.* 2011;38:586-593.

Leone FP, Timmerman D, Bourne T, Valentin L, Epstein E, Goldstein SR, Marret H, Parsons AK, Gull B, Istre O, Sepulveda W, Ferrazzi E, Van den Bosch T. Terms, definitions and measurements to describe the sonographic features of the endometrium and intrauterine lesions: a consensus opinion from the International Endometrial Tumor Analysis (IETA) group. *Ultrasound Obstet Gynecol.* 2010;35:103-112.

Van den Bosch T, Coosemans A, Morina M, Timmerman D, Amant F. Screening for uterine tumours. *Best Pract Res Clin Obstet Gynaecol.* 2012;26:257-266.

E

Endometrial Hyperplasia and the Differential Diagnosis for Thick Endometrium

Synonyms/Description
Endometrial proliferation

Etiology
Endometrial hyperplasia refers to abnormal proliferation of endometrial glands and stroma, representing a spectrum of endometrial abnormalities ranging from benign overgrowth to precancerous tissue. Endometrial hyperplasia can cause a diffusely thickened endometrium or, less commonly, focal thickening within the cavity.

Ultrasound Findings
The sonographic appearance of endometrial hyperplasia is a heterogeneous thickening of the endometrial echo (lining). Endometrial hyperplasia may be circumferential, involving most of the endometrium or focal and nodular. In premenopausal patients, optimal evaluation of the endometrium is in the early follicular (proliferative) phase when the lining is at its thinnest. Later in the menstrual cycle the endometrium becomes topographically irregular, and the appearance of endometrial hyperplasia may be indistinguishable from the normal thickening that occurs during the luteal (secretory) phase. There are no established values for the normal width of the endometrial echo in premenopausal women. The sonographic texture of the endometrial echo is an important feature, and focal irregularities may be further delineated with sonohysterography.

In postmenopausal patients with bleeding, the normal width of the endometrium in longitudinal view should measure less than or equal to 4 mm and appear linear, with no focal irregularities. Some authors report that a measurement less than 5 mm is normal; hence there is disagreement as to whether the upper limit of normal should be 4 or 5 mm; however, the American College of Obstetrics and Gynecology states less than or equal to 4 mm is normal. It is important to evaluate the endometrium in its entirety. If part of the endometrium is obscured by fibroids, polyps, or adenomyosis or if the margins are indistinct, saline infusion sonohysterography can be used for further evaluation. There is no accepted normative data for the width of the endometrium in nonbleeding postmenopausal patients. The sonographic appearance of the endometrial echo and color flow are important factors in detecting the presence of endometrial disease.

Tamoxifen is a selective estrogen receptor modulator used in the treatment and prevention of breast cancer. The estrogen receptor agonist activity in the uterus caused by Tamoxifen has been associated with an increased risk of endometrial polyps, hyperplasia, and cancer when used in postmenopausal women. In addition, patients on Tamoxifen can have a very indistinct endometrial/myometrial border that often results in the overestimation of the endometrial echo width. This is often caused by microcystic formation in the subendometrial region, which results in an irregular endometrial-myometrial junction. These microcysts are glandular cystic atrophy. Sonohysterography is very useful to delineate the true appearance of the endometrial surface itself.

Differential Diagnosis
The differential diagnosis for a thickened endometrium is extensive, but generally includes endometrial hyperplasia, polyps, fibroids (submucous),

endometrial cancer, retained products of conception, and adenomyosis. Patients with endometrial hyperplasia typically have a circumferentially thickened endometrium. Unfortunately, endometrial hyperplasia and cancer are indistinguishable sonographically and require tissue sampling.

Sonohysterography is crucial to differentiating a focal lesion such as a polyp from a global process such as hyperplasia or malignancy. Polyps are echogenic focal lesions, typically with a feeder vessel, and often detectable without sonohysterography. Submucous fibroids are typically rounded structures, more echolucent than the surrounding endometrium and displacing the endometrial echo. Adenomyosis may make the endometrial-myometrial junction indistinct, necessitating a sonohysterogram to clarify. If a patient has had a recent pregnancy, retained products of conception should be considered. Color flow Doppler may show extensive vascularity, further confirming the diagnosis. Please see the individual sections for Endometrial Carcinoma; Polyps, Endometrial; Adenomyosis; and Retained Products of Conception for more detail on each.

Clinical Aspects and Recommendations

Clinically there is a great difference between endometrial evaluation in premenopausal and postmenopausal patients. In premenopausal patients who are still cycling, it is essential that sonographic evaluation be performed in the early follicular phase, when the endometrium is thinnest. In postmenopausal patients who are not on hormone therapy, there is no "cycling," and sonographic evaluation may be carried out at any time. The value of sonography in patients suspected of having endometrial hyperplasia is the high negative predicative value of a thin, distinct endometrial echo when present. When a thin echo is not present, saline infusion sonohysterography can help to differentiate between global abnormalities, which can be sampled blindly, and focal abnormalities (polyps, focal tissue growth), which should be sampled under direct visualization (hysteroscopically).

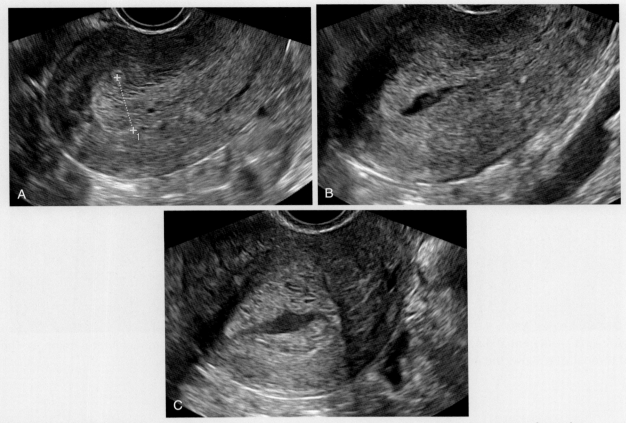

Figure E3-1 Endometrial hyperplasia. **A,** A diffusely thickened endometrium. **B and C,** Images from the sonohysterogram showing that the thickening is global.

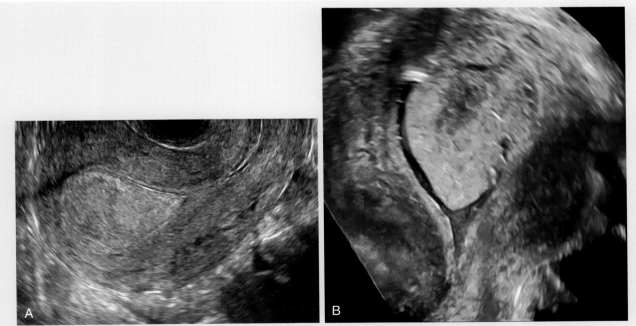

Figure E3-2 Differential diagnosis. **A,** A thickened endometrium. **B,** A 3-D image from the sonohysterogram showing a focal lesion that was a large polyp.

E

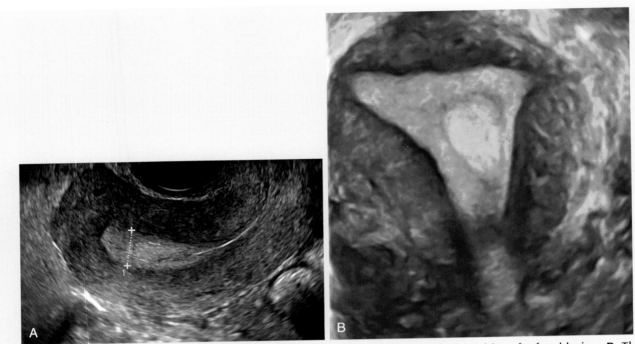

Figure E3-3   Differential diagnosis. **A,** A thickened and blotchy endometrium with a hint of a focal lesion. **B,** The 3-D coronal view shows the polyp without the need for a sonohysterogram.

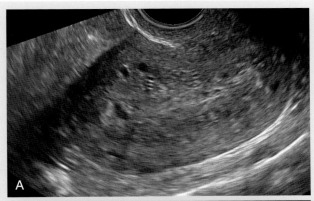

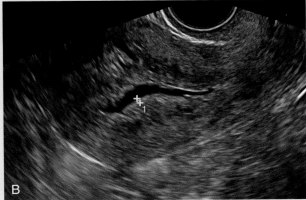

Figure E3-4 Differential diagnosis. **A,** A thick and irregular endometrium with many cystic spaces obscuring the endometrial-myometrial junction. This patient was on Tamoxifen, and the ultrasound image was not sufficient to evaluate the endometrium. **B,** The sonohysterogram, which revealed that most of the cystic areas are in the subendometrial region.

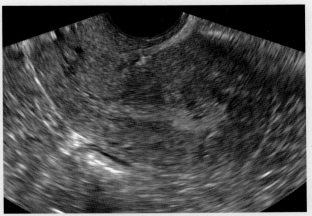

Figure E3-5 Differential diagnosis. Longitudinal view of the endometrium of a postmenopausal patient with bleeding. Note the focal nodular thickening of the endometrium at the fundus (retroverted uterus), with slight irregularity and loss of definition of the endometrial-myometrial junction. The pathology revealed papillary serous adenocarcinoma of the endometrium.

Suggested Reading

Ballard P, Tetlow R, Richmond I, Killick S, Purdie DW. Errors in the measurement of endometrial depth using transvaginal sonography in postmenopausal women on tamoxifen: random error is reduced using saline instillation sonography. *Ultrasound Obstet Gynecol.* 2000;15:321-326.

Goldstein RB, Bree RL, Benson CB, Benacerraf BR, Bloss JD, Carlos R, Fleischer AC, Goldstein SR, Hunt RB, Kurman RJ, Kurtz AB, Laing FC, Parsons AK, Smith-Bindman R, Walker J. Evaluation of the woman with postmenopausal bleeding: Society of Radiologists in Ultrasound-Sponsored Consensus Conference statement. *J Ultrasound Med.* 2001;20:1025-1036.

Goldstein SR. Modern evaluation of the endometrium. *Obstet Gynecol.* 2010;116:168-176.

Goldstein SR. Significance of incidentally thick endometrial echo on transvaginal ultrasound in postmenopausal women. *Menopause.* 2011;18:434-436.

Goldstein SR. Sonography in postmenopausal bleeding. *J Ultrasound Med.* 2012;31:333-336.

Mills AM, Longacre TA. Endometrial hyperplasia. *Semin Diagn Pathol.* 2010;27:199-214.

Montgomery BE, Daum GS, Dunton CJ. Endometrial hyperplasia: a review. *Obstet Gynecol Surv.* 2004;59(5):368-378.

E

Endometriosis

Synonyms/Description

Endometriosis signifies the presence of endometrial tissue outside the endometrial cavity. These ectopic glands respond to the cyclical hormones, thus causing microscopic internal bleeding and pain during the course of the menstrual cycle. This ectopic tissue bleeds episodically, causing inflammation, adhesions, and scarring. These ectopic glands can also react to hormones of pregnancy.

Etiology

The exact cause of endometriosis is unknown and there are multiple theories. In addition, the true prevalence of this condition is also unclear because endometriosis is not always symptomatic. There does, however, appear to be a higher incidence in women who are diagnosed with infertility and pelvic pain.

Endometriosis can occur in many forms, including the formation of cysts known as endometriomas (chocolate cysts), which typically develop in ovarian tissue. Endometriosis can also occur in the uterus with the propagation of endometrial glands through the junctional zone into the myometrium, a condition known as adenomyosis (see Adenomyosis). Endometriosis can also take the form of small deep implants of endometrial tissue in many different places in the body, including the wall of the bladder, the anterior abdominal wall, the bowel wall, and the uterosacral ligaments, as well as other pelvic sites. Rarely, endometriosis can occur in distal sites such as the lung, potentially causing hemoptysis.

Ultrasound Findings
Endometrioma

The typical appearance of an endometrioma is that of a unilocular cyst with homogeneous low-level echoes and through transmission of sound.

The ground-glass texture of the cyst content is very characteristic and makes 90% of endometriomas easily recognizable. Some benign endometriomas also have solid components (often echogenic) in the inner aspect of the cysts, but these are typically without discernible blood flow and represent clot. When interrogating endometriomas with color Doppler, there is no discernible flow in the cyst (only in the wall) and there is usually no visible streaming of the low-level echoes within the cyst, thus distinguishing it from cystadenomas and other cysts. Patients with endometriomas often have adhesions so that tubal disease in the form of a hydrosalpinx or other signs of adhesive disease may be a common finding.

When the cyst wall is thickened and irregular, the possibility of malignancy, specifically endometrioid carcinoma, must be considered. Typically endometrioid carcinoma looks like an endometrioma but with internal solid nodularity that contains abundant color Doppler flow. In a study of 309 endometrioid cysts surgically removed, 1.2% were classified as borderline, and 3.4% as invasive endometrioid tumors. Patients with malignancies were typically older (median 52 years) compared with those with benign cysts (median 34 years). All of the malignant and borderline tumors were characterized as having solid components with evidence of color flow, compared with only 7.8% of the benign lesions.

Decidualized Endometrioma

If the patient is pregnant, the endometrioma may become decidualized and have ultrasound characteristics suggestive of a malignancy. The stromal transformation of endometrial cells within the endometrioma can occur because of high levels of progesterone in pregnancy. In gravid patients, these cysts can contain internal solid nodularity with blood flow, and are indistinguishable from borderline or even frank ovarian cancers sonographically.

Therefore such cysts may potentially be watched with frequent serial ultrasounds before making a final decision to remove the cyst during the pregnancy. If the cyst remains unchanged, it is unlikely to be malignant, and removal can be planned after delivery.

Deep Penetrating Bowel Wall and Pelvic Implants

Sonographically, deep implants of endometriosis are small solid masses with little if any detectable blood flow using color Doppler. The bowel wall implants are nodular and fusiform swellings of one side of the bowel wall. This swelling is often adherent to the back of the cervix, thus hindering any sliding of the uterus past the bowel on exam. Bazot reports a sensitivity and specificity of 78.5% and 95.2%, respectively, for detecting disease in that location, suggesting that ultrasound (in experienced hands) is accurate in diagnosing rectosigmoid endometriosis. Hudelist and colleagues report a sensitivity and specificity of 91% and 98%, respectively, and positive likelihood ratio and negative likelihood ratios of 30.4 and 0.1, respectively, for detecting bowel wall endometriosis using ultrasound. Although MRI can also detect implants of endometriosis, evidence shows that pain-guided transvaginal ultrasound is likely more sensitive for detecting bowel involvement.

Implants in the rectovaginal septum are also nodular, small, rounded, solid structures best seen along the most distal portion of the cervix and along the posterior fornix and upper vagina. Implants may also be found on the pelvic ligaments such as the uterosacral ligaments and para pelvic regions.

Bladder Wall, Ureter, and Anterior Abdominal Wall Lesions (Also See Bladder Masses)

Implants of endometriosis can occur practically anywhere; however, the more common areas of involvement include the bladder wall, ureter, and anterior abdominal wall in patients who have had abdominal surgery such as a prior C-section or laparoscopy. Endometriosis of the bladder wall appears as a fusiform solid thickening of the wall itself. If endometrial implants impinge on the ureter, the patient may have chronic ureteral obstruction that is silent and may lead to a nonfunctioning kidney.

In patients who have had prior abdominal surgery, endometriosis may present as a hard, solid mass in the anterior abdominal wall in the region of the scar. Little color flow may be present, and the mass is often tender.

Differential Diagnosis
Endometrioma

Most endometriomas involve the ovary and have a characteristic appearance, which is a unilocular cyst with homogeneous low-level echoes and no color flow. Some endometriomas can be multilocular or septate or have a thickened wall with echogenic material. These cysts may be confused with dermoids (echogenic area), cystadenomas (septations), or even malignancy if there is some solid component. Color Doppler is essential to interrogate these solid areas for blood flow. The absence of flow may suggest a cystadenoma-fibroma or endometrioma. If color flow is present, one must consider decidualized endometrioma (in pregnancy) versus a borderline or invasive endometrioid carcinoma.

Streaming is typically absent in endometriomas when using Doppler. If the cyst has streaming echoes, a diagnosis other than endometriosis should be considered.

Deep Penetrating Bowel Wall and Pelvic Implants

Patients with deep bowel wall and pelvic endometrial implants are typically in a lot of pain during the transvaginal examination, and the pelvic organs tend to be adherent to each other. It is important to try to move the uterus with the vaginal probe to see if it slides past the anterior wall of the rectosigmoid and the ovaries. If these organs are stuck together in a patient with pain, then endometriosis is likely. Other lesions involving the bowel wall include inflammatory bowel disease or lymphoma; however, both of these diseases have diffuse (nonfocal) bowel involvement without extensive adhesions or focal pain (see Bowel Diseases). Solid implants with color flow in the peritoneal cavity may indicate carcinomatosis, although this is usually accompanied by ascites.

Bladder Wall Lesions

Endometriosis of the bladder wall is usually well contained within the wall and has little detectable blood flow. The mucosal surface remains smooth, unlike a transitional cell carcinoma, which is a fungating vascular lesion of the mucosal surface.

Clinical Aspects and Recommendations

The three general categories that comprise the clinical manifestations of endometriosis include (1) pelvic pain, (2) infertility, and (3) pelvic mass. The goal of any therapy is to relieve the symptoms. There are so many different medical treatments that decisions regarding management must be individualized, taking into account severity of symptoms, extent and location of the disease, desire for future fertility, medication side effects, surgical complication rates, and even cost.

Detailed treatment options are beyond the scope of this section, but would include expectant management, analgesia, various hormonal medical therapies, surgical intervention, which may be conservative and tissue sparing or definitive (total abdominal hysterectomy and possible bilateral salpingo-oophorectomy), or combinations of these therapies. As always,

minimally invasive surgery in the form of laparoscopy would be preferable to open laparotomy although often the extent of adhesions may make a minimally invasive approach difficult, if not impossible.

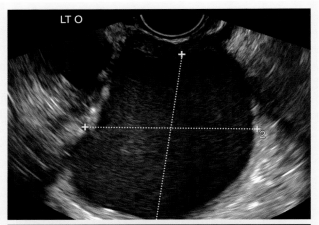

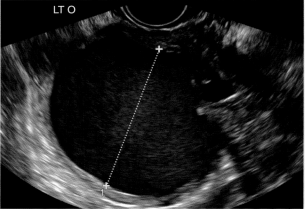

Figure E4-1   Two views of a left ovarian endometrioma. Note the typical ground-glass sonographic texture of the cyst contents with a slightly irregular wall.

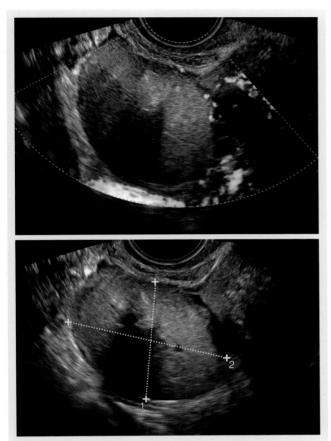

Figure E4-2 Two views of an endometrioma involving the right ovary. Note that the internal texture is mixed with a hyperechoic area with shadowing, which may suggest a dermoid cyst in the differential diagnosis.

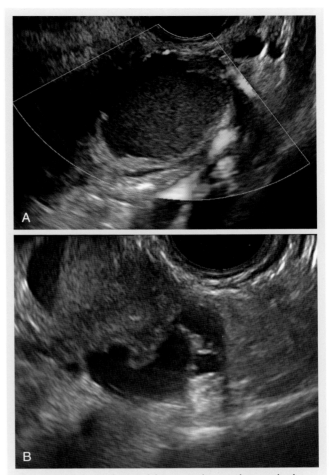

Figure E4-4 Patient with extensive endometriosis. **A,** A typical endometrioma with a thick and irregular wall but no color flow demonstrated. **B,** The associated hydrosalpinx adjacent to the cyst.

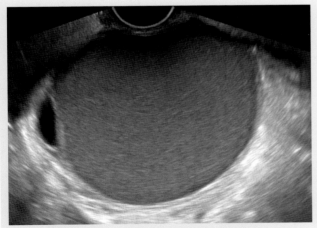

Figure E4-3 Typical unilocular endometrioma. The small, clear cyst compressed on one side is likely a follicle.

E

E

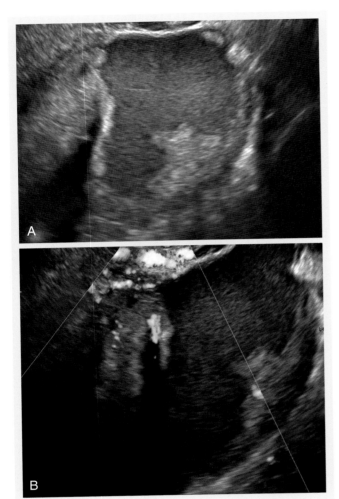

A

B

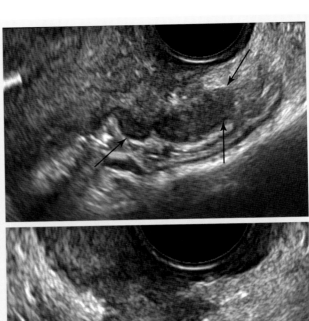

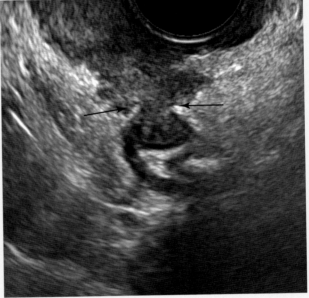

Figure E4-5 **A,** Cystic mass in a pregnant patient showing an irregular and nodular inner wall with cystic contents displaying low-level echoes. **B,** Image showing blood flow in the solid areas, a finding that is worrisome for a malignancy. This mass was proved to be a decidualized endometrioma at surgery.

Figure E4-6 Transverse and longitudinal views of the anterior wall of the rectosigmoid, showing solid nodular masses compressing the lumen *(arrows)*. These are typical of endometriotic implants in the bowel wall. Note that the involved bowel is adjacent to the back of the cervix and posterior fornix of the vagina.

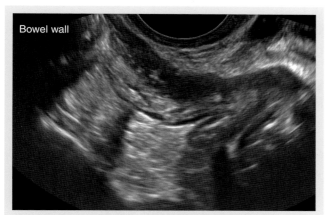

Figure E4-7   Long segment of sigmoid involved with endometriosis of the bowel wall on one side. Note the asymmetric thickening of the anterior wall.

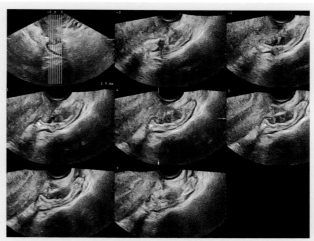

Figure E4-9   Three-dimensional multislide view of the affected bowel wall showing the involved bowel segment adjacent to the back of the cervix (cephalad).

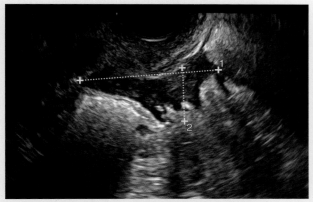

Figure E4-8   Focal area of involvement of the rectovaginal septum, showing the typical fingerlike projections from the nodular wall toward the lumen of the rectum. The rectum, upper vagina, and cervix were all adhered to each other, and the area was very tender during the scan.

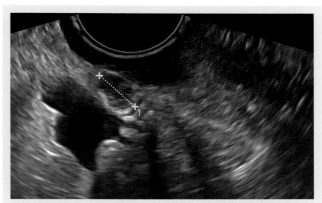

Figure E4-10   Small subcentimeter endometriotic implant along the posterior aspect of the cervix. Note that the free fluid in the cul-de-sac appears on the outside of the implant rather than directly adjacent to the cervix.

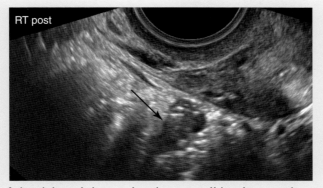

Figure E4-11   Oblique view of the right cul-de-sac showing a small implant on the utero-sacral ligament in a patient with extensive disease. This lesion was very tender.

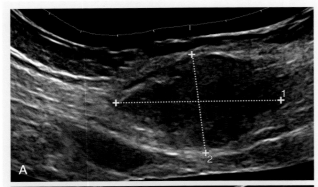

Figure E4-12 Fusiform thickening of the bladder wall in a patient with endometriosis of the bladder.

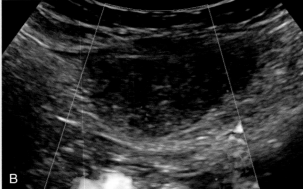

Figure E4-13 Two views of a solid and tender lesion in the anterior abdominal wall within a C-section scar. **B,** A paucity of blood flow in the mass, typical of endometriosis.

Videos
Videos 1, 2, 3, 4, and 5 on endometriosis/endometrioma are available online.

Suggested Reading
Koninckx PR, Ussia A, Adamyan L, Wattiez A, Donnez J. Deep endometriosis: definition, diagnosis, and treatment. *Fertil Steril.* 2012;98:564-571.

Miranda-Mendoza I, Kovoor E, Nassif J, Ferreira H, Wattiez A. Laparoscopic surgery for severe ureteric endometriosis. *Eur J Obstet Gynecol Reprod Biol.* 2012 Dec; 165(2):275-279.

Ozel L, Sagiroglu J, Unal A, Unal E, Gunes P, Baskent E, Aka N, Titiz MI, Tufekci EC. Abdominal wall endometriosis in the cesarean section surgical scar: a potential diagnostic pitfall. *J Obstet Gynaecol Res.* 2012;38:526-530.

Poder L, Coakley FV, Rabban JT, Goldstein RB, Aziz S, Chen LM. Decidualized endometrioma during pregnancy: recognizing an imaging mimic of ovarian malignancy. *J Comput Assist Tomogr.* 2008;32:555-558.

Testa AC, Timmerman D, Van Holsbeke C, Zannoni GF, Fransis S, Moerman P, Vellone V, Mascilini F, Licameli A, Ludovisi M, Di Legge A, Scambia G, Ferrandina G. Ovarian cancer arising in endometrioid cysts: ultrasound findings. *Ultrasound Obstet Gynecol.* 2011;38:99-106.

Epidermoid Cyst

Synonyms/Description

Epidermal cyst or sebaceous cyst of the ovary
Mature monophyletic teratoma

Etiology

Epidermoid cysts are benign cysts, lined by mature keratinizing squamous epithelium but without hair (unlike dermoids). These lesions represent less than 0.25% of all ovarian neoplasms. Two main theories exist regarding the etiology: This may be a monophyletic variant of a dermoid or teratoma with only the epithelial component present, resulting in a highly differentiated lesion. Alternatively, epidermoid cysts may arise from epithelial cell nests in the ovary similar to those seen in Brenner tumors. The cysts can contain keratin and other sebaceous material. There is a similar counterpart tumor that occurs in the testes.

Ultrasound Findings

Epidermoid cysts are solid-appearing lesions with heterogeneous and echogenic texture but no internal color flow on Doppler evaluation. The detectable blood flow is peripheral, suggesting a cyst wall. Epidermoid cysts are not as echogenic as dermoids, making the appearance nonspecific. The lack of flow inside is helpful in this otherwise solid-appearing lesion.

Differential Diagnosis

The presence of a solid ovarian mass brings to mind many diagnoses. The lack of internal blood flow typical of the epidermoid cyst helps to narrow the differential diagnoses to dermoid, endometrioma, fibroma, or other benign solid ovarian tumor.

Clinical Aspects and Recommendations

Epidermoid cyst is usually detected as an incidental finding on a pathology specimen, benign, and rarely symptomatic.

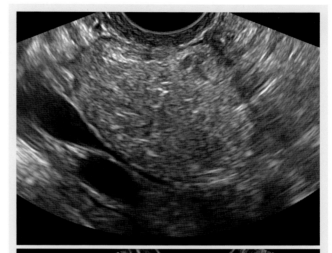
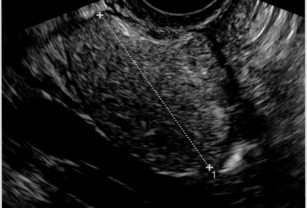

Figure E5-1 Two views of an ovarian epidermoid cyst. Note the slightly echogenic but heterogeneous internal sonographic texture.

E

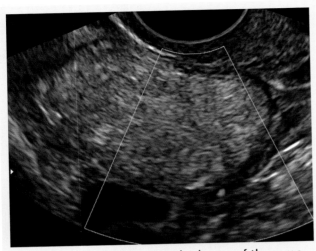

Figure E5-2   Color flow Doppler image of the same epidermoid cyst showing only peripheral flow in the capsule of the cyst.

Suggested Reading

Fan LD, Zang HY, Zhang XS. Ovarian epidermoid cyst: report of eight cases. *Int J Gynecol Pathol.* 1996;15:69-71.

Sheikh SS, Amr SS. Epidermoid cyst of the ovary. *J Obstet Gynaecol.* 2003;23:213.

E

Fibroids

Synonyms/Description
Leiomyoma, myoma, fibromyoma, and uterine fibroma

Etiology
Fibroids are the most common benign pelvic tumor in women. The prevalence in women age 50 and older is estimated at 80% in African Americans and up to 70% in Caucasians. Others have estimated a lower incidence (up to 50% of perimenopausal women).

Myomas are thought to be monoclonal and originate from a single myocyte that undergoes somatic mutation as it grows. Cytogenetic anomalies are found in 40% of fibroids. Estrogen and progesterone are known to stimulate the growth of fibroids. Although many fibroids are asymptomatic, others may cause bleeding, pain, mass effect, urinary frequency, constipation, pregnancy loss, and infertility. The presence of symptomatic fibroids is the most common indication for hysterectomy.

Ultrasound Findings
Fibroids are typically solid masses, which are sonographically hypoechoic or isoechoic with the surrounding myometrium. They are well circumscribed, with acoustic shadowing, often with a pattern of stripes or swirls caused by these shadows. They can be calcified, often with a circumferential pattern of calcification. If they degenerate, they can have central cystic portions. Color Doppler findings of fibroids are variable. Some fibroids have abundant flow and others scant; therefore there is no Doppler flow pattern specific to fibroids. Doppler is helpful to map the blood flow to the fibroid. If it is pedunculated, it may be confused with an ovarian mass.

Fibroids are further described by their location in the uterus.

Intramural
Fibroids are most commonly intramural and occur within the confines of myometrium.

Submucosal
A fibroid that protrudes into the endometrial cavity is submucosal. These can occasionally be pedunculated into the cavity and slide down into the cervix as the uterus tries to expel it. Three-dimensional ultrasound and sonohysterography can be very helpful in outlining the extent of the submucosal component of the fibroid within the cavity.

Subserosal
A fibroid that indents the serosal surface and gives a bumpy appearance of the outside of the uterus is subserosal.

Pedunculated
A fibroid that has grown from a subserosal fibroid outward and remains tethered to the uterus by a pedicle is considered pedunculated. Occasionally these can pick up vascularity from outside organs and become parasitic, no longer connected to the uterus, making the sonographic diagnosis more difficult.

Degenerating
Discrepancy between the rate of growth of the myoma and its blood supply can lead to an infarction of part (most often the center) of the myoma. The degenerating fibroid has a variable manifestation, the most common being a donut-appearing mass with a cystic center and a thick wall, located within the confines of the uterus. The acute infarction leads to severe pain and is more common during pregnancy. Some degenerating fibroids can mimic ovarian cystic masses, especially if they are pedunculated and multiseptate in appearance.

Differential Diagnosis

The differential diagnosis of fibroids depends on the location and appearance of the uterine mass. A fibroid that contains cystic areas and abundant blood flow may be indistinguishable sonographically from a uterine sarcoma (see Sarcoma). Follow-up scans showing aggressive growth, particularly in a postmenopausal patient, would suggest a malignancy. If the mass is ill-defined, it may represent an adenomyoma, which is similar in appearance to a fibroid, but has blurry or indistinct borders and is often seen in a setting of adenomyosis (see Endometriosis). If the fibroid is submucosal and more echogenic than usual, it could be confused with an endometrial polyp. A central blood supply with a feeding vessel and cystic spaces would favor a polyp. A bumpy and asymmetric uterus may be confused with a Müllerian duct anomaly such as a unicornuate uterus with a rudimentary horn forming a mass. Three-dimensional ultrasound is essential for diagnosing Müllerian duct abnormalities and the position of fibroids within the uterus.

If the fibroid is pedunculated laterally, in the broad ligament, it may be difficult to distinguish it from a solid adnexal mass such as a fibroma or Brenner tumor. Finding the ipsilateral ovary separate from the mass is important to rule out such entities.

Clinical Aspects and Recommendations

Fibroids are so common and variable in size and location that clinical management and recommendations depend on many variables, such as age, parity, desire for future fertility, bleeding pattern, and hormonal status (e.g., premenopausal vs. postmenopausal). In general, therapies for fibroids include gonadotropin-releasing hormone agonists, hysterectomy or myomectomy (abdominal or transcervical), MRI-guided focused ultrasound surgery, and uterine artery embolization. Symptom severity and a desire to maintain uterine preservation are factors in determining treatment choice.

In patients desiring future fertility, uterine preservation is crucial, and either expectant management or conservative surgery (myomectomy) is employed. Increasingly, minimally invasive techniques (transcervical resection, morcellation for selected submucous myomas, or laparoscopic surgery) would be preferred over traditional open abdominal myomectomy. Conservative management of bleeding can often be accomplished hormonally with combination contraceptives (pills, patch, or vaginal ring), the levonorgestrel-releasing IUD, progestin-only pills, tranexamic acid, and even nonsteroidal anti-inflammatory drugs (NSAIDs) in some patients. Preoperatively, GnRH agonists such as leuprolide or danazol have been employed to reduce uterine size. Some women close to menopause may use such agents to eliminate bleeding and reduce uterine size, thus allowing them to drift into natural menopause, when symptoms and bleeding will cease. In patients with severe symptoms of pelvic pressure, pain, bowel/bladder complaints, or abnormal uterine bleeding, hysterectomy will be definitive therapy. Other less invasive approaches such as high-frequency focused ultrasound (HiFUS) and uterine artery embolization are also used.

Perimenopausal patient's estradiol levels initially rise as women become anovulatory and produce multiple follicles, without any becoming dominant. This can result in temporary enlargement of fibroids before actual menopause and may concern clinicians. Although uterine sarcomas may be difficult to distinguish sonographically from very vascular fibroids, true leiomyomas are benign and do not undergo malignant degeneration.

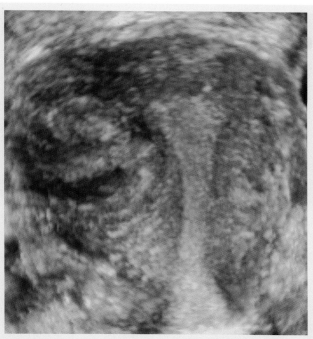

Figure F1-1   3-D ultrasound showing an intramural fibroid in the right midbody of the uterus.

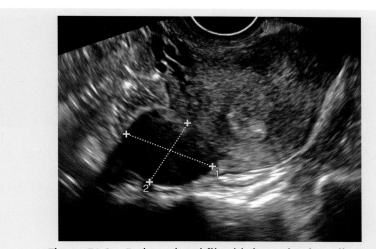

Figure F1-2   Pedunculated fibroid shown by the calipers.

F

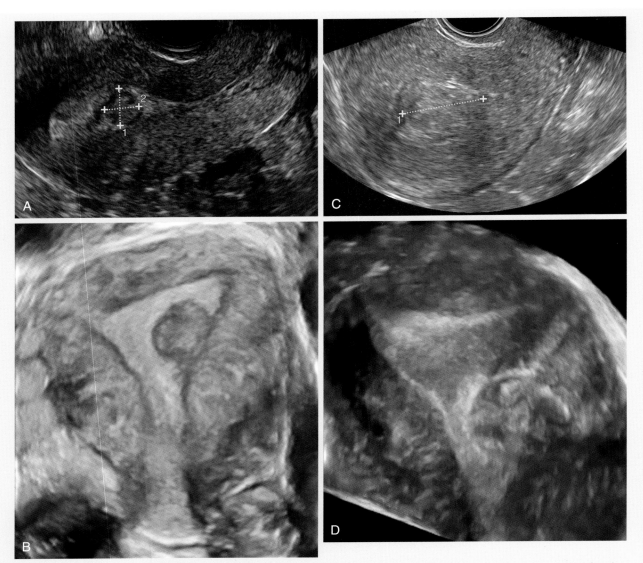

Figure F1-3 Two cases of submucosal fibroids (2-D and 3-D coronal views). **A and B,** Small, almost completely submucosal fibroid in the left side of the cavity best seen with 3-D. **C and D,** Larger fibroid, lower in the uterus and 50% submucoal. Three-dimensional imaging is necessary to map out the exact position of the fibroid within the uterine cavity.

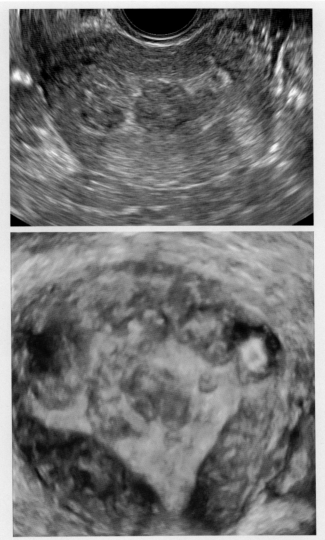

Figure F1-4   2-D and 3-D views of multiple submucoal fibroids throughout the uterus.

F

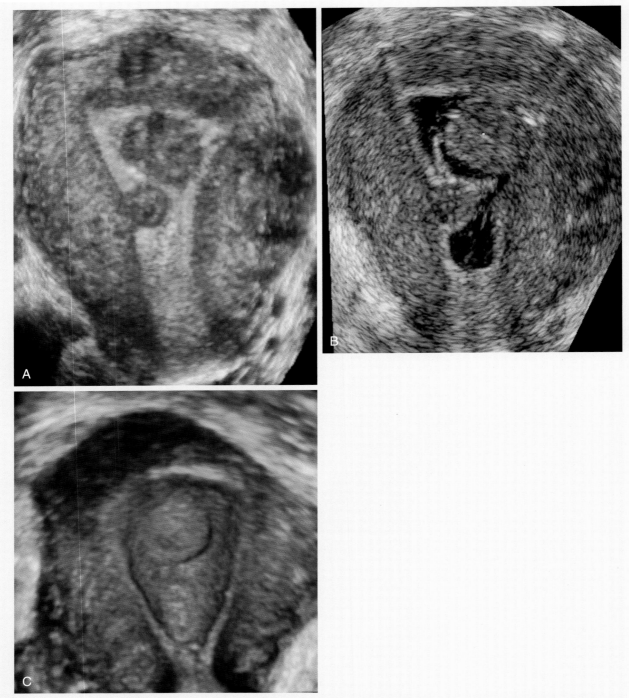

Figure F1-5 Submucosal fibroids using sonohysterography for mapping. **A,** Simple 3-D coronal view. **B,** After instilling saline into the cavity. **C,** Virtual hysteroscopy using the 3-D surface view.

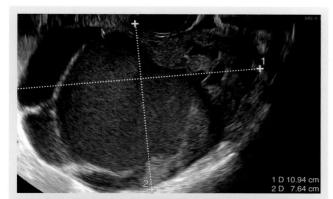

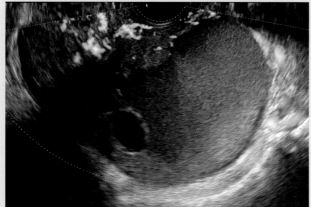

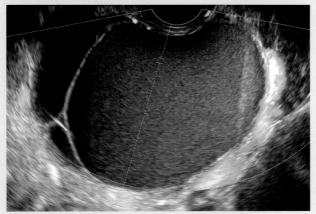

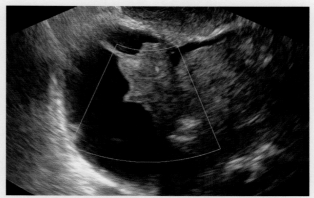

Figure F1-7 Another case of a degenerating fibroid showing very little blood flow. Note the uterus on the right, adjacent to the mass.

Figure F1-6 Degenerating fibroid: Multiseptate mass with peripheral blood flow. This atypical appearance could be confused with an ovarian tumor or an endometrioma. Finding a separate ovary as well as a connection between the mass and the uterus is essential to make the correct diagnosis.

F

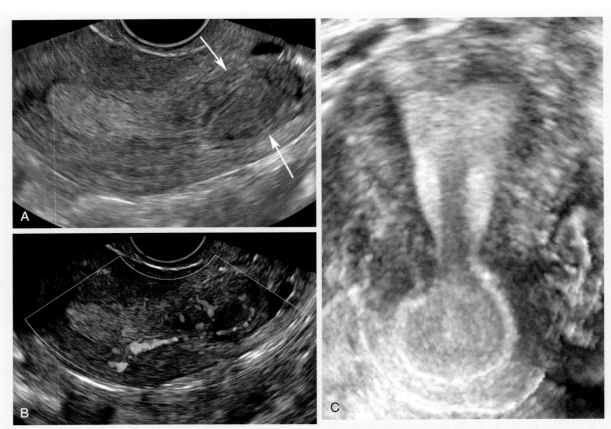

Figure F1-8 **A,** Pedunculated submucosal fibroid prolapsing through the cervix *(arrows)*. **B,** Color Doppler shows feeding vessels. **C,** 3-D coronal view shows the position of the fibroid.

Suggested Reading

American College of Obstetricians and Gynecologists. Alternatives to hysterectomy in the management of leiomyomas. ACOG Practice Bulletin No. 96. *Obstet Gynecol.* 2008;112:201.

Evans P, Brunsell S. Uterine fibroid tumors: diagnosis and treatment. *Am Fam Physician.* 2007;75:1503-1508.

Flake GP, Andersen J, Dixon D. Etiology and pathogenesis of uterine leiomyomas: a review. *Environ Health Perspect.* 2003;111:1037-1054.

Levy BS. Modern management of uterine fibroids. *Acta Obstet Gynecol Scand.* 2008;87:812-823.

Parker WH. Uterine myomas: management. *Fertil Steril.* 2007;88:255-271.

Stewart EA. Uterine fibroids. *Lancet.* 2001;357:293.

Vitiello D, McCarthy S. Diagnostic imaging of myomas. *Obstet Gynecol Clin North Am.* 2006:3385-3395.

Fibroma (Ovarian), Thecoma, and Fibrothecoma

Synonyms/Description

Thecoma, fibroma, and fibrothecoma are all tumors belonging to the thecoma-fibroma group of stromal tumors (per the World Health Organization classification of ovarian sex cord–stromal tumors).

Etiology

Thecoma-fibroma tumors are a closely related group of benign tumors that arise from ovarian stroma and are often difficult for the imager and even pathologist to distinguish. The fibroma contains spindle cells, and is the most common type of sex cord-stromal tumor, accounting for 6% of all ovarian tumors. They are usually asymptomatic although they can be large.

The thecoma arises from theca (stroma) cells and can produce estrogen, much like the granulosa cell tumors, thus sometimes presenting with abnormal uterine bleeding. Many of these tumors are a mixture of cell types and are called fibrothecoma.

Ultrasound Findings

Fibromas/thecomas are typically solid, rounded, or oval ovarian lesions and may attain a large size (fibroma) and have low to moderate vascularity. Sonographically, fibromas tend to cast an intense acoustic shadow, making it difficult to see beyond the anterior surface of the tumor. They can also be solid but "stripy," with linear streaks appearing vertically within the lesion. Vascularity is typically low by color Doppler, but occasional lesions may be more vascular, such as cellular fibromas. There can be small cystic areas within the solid mass; however, large cystic components are extremely rare.

Differential Diagnosis

These solid tumors cast intense acoustic shadows either as stripes or simply a global shadow from the entire lesion. A pedunculated fibroid is the most likely differential diagnosis to mimic this appearance. The finding of a normal ovary separate from the solid tumor can help to make that differentiation. Other solid ovarian tumors such as teratomas, dysgerminomas, and some solid malignancies are unlikely to cast a shadow and tend to be more vascular throughout the lesion than the fibroma/thecoma.

Clinical Aspects and Recommendations

Larger lesions are sometimes associated with ascites and rarely even hydrothorax. Meigs' syndrome (ascites and hydrothorax) occurs in 10% of all cases and 40% of the time when the tumor exceeds 10 cm in diameter.

Similar to myomas they can sometimes have increased mitotic figures per 10 high-powered fields. True ovarian fibrothecomas, however, are extremely rare. Treatment generally consists of salpingo-oophorectomy. Occasionally, because thecomas can produce estrogen and present with postmenopausal bleeding, endometrial sampling is indicated.

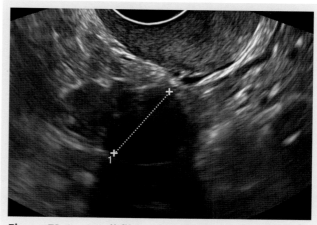

Figure F2-1 Small fibroma indicated by the calipers. The lesion is almost invisible due to the intense acoustic shadow cast by the front of the mass.

F

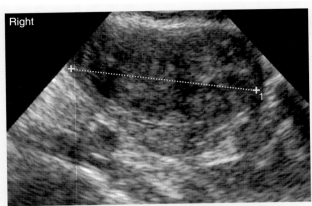

Figure F2-2 Fibroma—typically oval, completely solid but smooth mass.

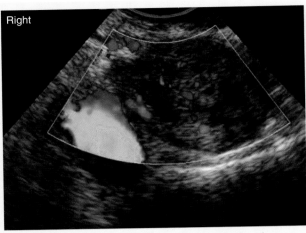

Figure F2-4 Fibroma with more vascularity than usually seen.

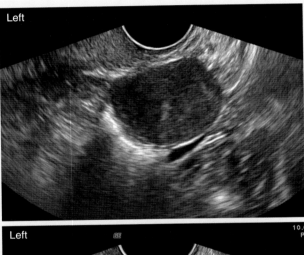

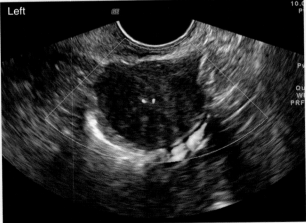

Figure F2-3 Fibrothecoma with and without Doppler flow showing a typical solid mass with internal shadowing and limited vascularity.

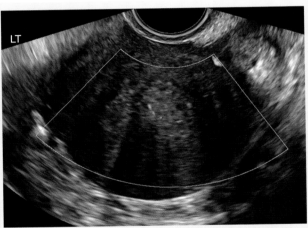

Figure F2-5 Large fibroma with limited Doppler color flow and linear vertical shadows down the middle of the mass, typical of fibromas.

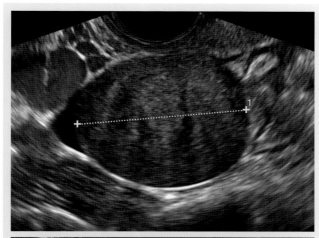

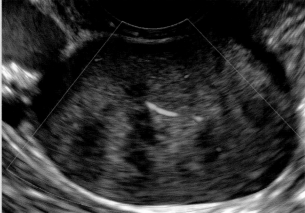

Figure F2-6 Fibroma presenting as a large solid ovarian mass in a pregnant woman. Note the multiple vertical linear stripes and poor vascularity of this mass.

Suggested Reading

Chechia A, Attia L, Temime RB, Makhlouf T, Koubaa A. Incidence, clinical analysis, and management of ovarian fibromas and fibrothecomas. *Am J Obstet Gynecol.* 2008;199:473.e1-4.

Conte M, Guariglia L, Benedetti Panici P, Scambia G, Rabitti C, Capelli A, Mancuso S. Ovarian fibrothecoma: sonographic and histologic findings. *Gynecol Obstet Invest.* 1991;32:51-54.

Paladini D, Testa A, Van Holsbeke C, Mancari R, Timmerman D, Valentin L. Imaging in gynecological disease (5): clinical and ultrasound characteristics in fibroma and fibrothecoma of the ovary. *Ultrasound Obstet Gynecol.* 2009;34:188-195.

Yaghoobian J, Pinck RL. Ultrasound findings in thecoma of the ovary. *J Clin Ultrasound.* 1983;11: 91-93.

Yen P, Khong K, Lamba R, Corwin MT, Gerscovich EO. Ovarian fibromas and fibrothecomas. *J Ultrasound Med.* 2013;32:13-18.

F

Granulosa Cell Tumor

Synonyms/Description
Granulosa-theca cell tumor
Sex cord–gonadal stromal tumor

Etiology
Granulosa cell tumors (GCTs) are relatively rare malignant neoplasms representing 3% of all ovarian cancers and 70% of tumors in the category of ovarian sex cord-stromal tumors. Granulosa cell tumors arise from a hormonally active component of the ovarian stroma that is responsible for estradiol production and hence represents 80% of hormone-producing ovarian tumors.

Granulosa cell tumor neoplasms are divided into the rare juvenile form (5%) and the more common adult type, which typically occurs in perimenopausal or postmenopausal women. The GCT is a slow-growing malignant tumor that typically spreads locally in the peritoneum and in 25% of patients recurs 5 to 10 years later, although sometimes decades after initial presentation.

Ultrasound Findings
Granulosa cell tumors can present as cystic/septated or solid masses arising from the ovary.

In the study by Van Holsbeke and colleagues, almost all tumors had solid components; 52% were multilocular with solid areas, 39% were purely solid, 4% were unilocular with a solid component, and 4% were multilocular. Granulosa cell tumors are typically large, with a median diameter of 10.2 cm (range, 3.7 to 24.2cm) in this study. Only one mass was smaller than 5 cm, and more than 50% were larger than 10 cm. Ascites was present in 22% of patients. Most of the tumors had a high vascular content shown by color Doppler, indicating a high likelihood of malignancy.

These tumors typically produce hyperestrogenemia, so patients are at increased risk for development of endometrial hyperplasia or concomitant endometrial adenocarcinoma. Sonographically, there may be evidence of a thickened endometrial lining.

Differential Diagnosis
Granulosa cell tumors are large tumors that can be solid, solid/cystic, and cystic with multiple septations. They tend to be large and associated with evidence of hyperestrogenemia such as abnormal bleeding. The differential diagnosis is vast and includes practically all large adnexal masses that contain septations, solid components, and vascularity. Other tumors such as epithelial malignancies can have a similar appearance. Fibromas tend to be predominantly solid with less blood flow than GCTs. Fibrothecomas are also solid in appearance and can produce estrogen, similar to the GCT.

Clinical Aspects and Recommendations
Postmenopausal or irregular bleeding is a common presenting sign in the adult form of GCT, likely because of exposure to estradiol, ultimately leading to endometrial hyperplasia or adenocarcinoma.

The juvenile type of GCT may present with precocious puberty or abdominal/pelvic pain as these can grow to large sizes.

The survival for GCT patients depends on staging. The 10-year survival rates for stages 1, 2, and 3/4 are 84% to 95%, 50% to 65%, and 17% to 33%, respectively. The management is surgical and depends on stage of disease.

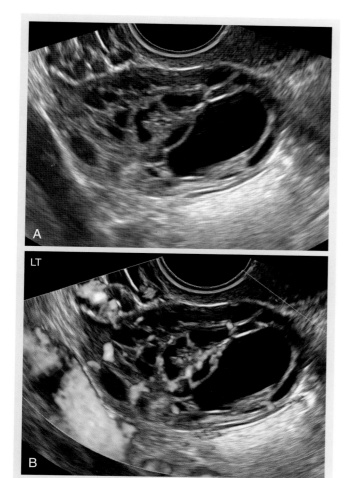

Figure G1-1 **A and B,** Large, heavily septated GCT with thick septae. **B,** The abundant vascularity in the thick septae.

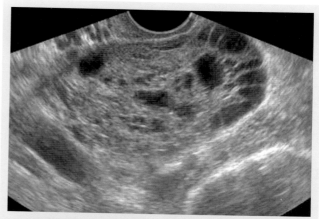

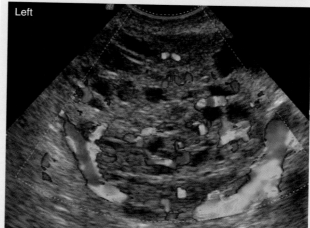

Figure G1-2 **A and B,** Large GCT with more solid portions than cystic. **B,** Note the intense vascularity on color Doppler.

Suggested Reading

Jung SE, Lee JM, Rha SE, Byun JY, Jung JI, Hahn ST. CT and MR imaging of ovarian tumors with emphasis on differential diagnosis. *Radiographics*. 2002;22:1305-1325.

Pectasides D, Pectasides E, Psyrri A. Granulosa cell tumor of the ovary. *Cancer Treat Rev.* 2008;34:1-12.

Schumer ST, Cannistra SA. Granulosa cell tumor of the ovary. *J Clin Oncol.* 2003;21:1180-1189.

G

Hematometra and Hematocolpos

Synonyms/Description
Hydrometra and hydrocolpos
Pyometra and pyocolpos

Etiology
The most common etiology is cervical or vaginal obstruction, resulting in a collection of blood, pus, or fluid that distends the uterus or vagina.

Hematometra/Hydrometra
Cervical stenosis can develop for multiple reasons (treatment for cervical dysplasia, prior ablation, postmenopausal effect), blocking the cervical canal and resulting in accumulation of fluid/blood in the uterine cavity. Advanced endometrial cancer can either block the canal or produce copious amounts of fluid/blood filling the uterine cavity. Many years ago, fluid in the endometrial cavity was considered a sonographic sign of cancer. More recently, Dr. Steven Goldstein showed that it is not the intracavitary fluid that conveys the risk of cancer, rather the appearance of the wall around the fluid. If the endometrium surrounding the fluid is smooth and thin, endometrial cancer is unlikely, whereas an irregular wall or mass protruding into the fluid indicates the presence of a tumor.

Benign causes of hematometra include an intracavitary fibroid or polyp in the cervix or lower uterine segment, and adhesions such as those encountered after an incomplete endometrial ablation. If the ablation seals the lower uterine segment but leaves intact endometrium at the fundus, cyclical hematometra with bilateral hematosalpinges may result. Patients with Müllerian duct anomalies who have a uterine duplication may have an obliterated horn, which will fill with blood and cause cyclical pain, typically presenting at puberty. This may pose a diagnostic dilemma if the uterine anomaly is not known, because these patients will present with a painful cystic mass in the pelvis often mistaken for a degenerating fibroid or adnexal mass. If the Müllerian duct anomaly is severe, the hematometra/hydrometra may even be visible prenatally as an intra-abdominal cystic mass in the fetus.

Hematocolpos/Hydrocolpos
Obstruction within the distal vagina is usually responsible for the development of a hematocolpos. If there is a backup of blood or fluid in the vagina, this may extend into the uterine cavity and result in an associated hematometra. Obstructions of the distal vagina are commonly owing to congenital Müllerian duct anomalies such as a transverse vaginal septum or an imperforate hymen. Patients with congenital anomalies of the vagina often have associated anomalies of the uterus; however, patients with vaginal obstruction may not become symptomatic until menarche.

Ultrasound Findings
The sonographic appearance of a hematometra/hydrometra is the presence of fluid distending the uterine cavity. Similarly hematocolpos/hydrocolpos is the presence of fluid in an obstructed vagina. The fluid often contains low-level echoes much like the texture of an endometrioma, indicating the presence of unclotted blood. The presence of more than a sliver of fluid in the uterus and/or vagina needs to be further investigated sonographically. Consider the patient's history: Has the patient had an ablation, and does she have cyclical symptoms? Is there a known Müllerian duct anomaly? Did the patient become symptomatic at menarche or is she asymptomatic? The ultrasound exam should include a 3-D evaluation of the uterine shape looking for Müllerian uterine anomalies (see Müllerian Duct Abnormalities). The tubes should be evaluated for the presence of fluid, to

H

determine if the obstruction has extended to the fallopian tubes. The inner lining of the uterus (endometrial surface) should be evaluated carefully for any masses indicating polyps or malignancy. The cervix should be assessed for the presence of obstructing lesions such as fibroids or large polyps. It may be difficult to see a small cervical carcinoma sonographically; however, the type of cervical lesion that obstructs the uterus is likely large enough to be visualized using a high-frequency transvaginal probe.

The vagina is often easier to evaluate sonographically by placing the vaginal probe on the introitus and looking down the length of the vagina and urethra (see Vaginal Masses and also Bladder Masses). Any fluid collection along the vagina may represent an obstructed hemivagina, a finding often associated with congenital uterine anomalies.

Differential Diagnosis

Fluid inside a normal uterine cavity does not have a differential diagnosis and is not always pathologic. It is important to note that a small amount of clear fluid in a postmenopausal uterus is not abnormal. The different causes of hematometra/hydrometra (described in Etiology, earlier) are the more diagnostically challenging step. The presence of fluid in an abnormal uterine cavity such as a rudimentary uterine horn can be confused with a cystic adnexal mass, including those of ovarian origin. If the ipsilateral ovary is normal sonographically, then fluid in a rudimentary horn may be confused with a degenerating fibroid or a hydrosalpinx. Recognizing the uterus as unicornuate using 3-D ultrasound would be an important clue to the correct diagnosis of a Müllerian duct abnormality. The presence of such a uterine anomaly is also vital to making the correct diagnosis of an obstructed hemivagina. Otherwise the vaginal fluid could be confused with a Gartner's duct cyst or urethral diverticulum (see Vaginal Masses and also Bladder Masses). The patient's age, pain, and menstruation history are likely to be important factors in arriving at the correct diagnosis.

Clinical Aspects and Recommendations

The cause of the hematometra/hydrometra or hematocolpos/hydrocolpos will guide the management. Patients who are asymptomatic and simply have a small amount of clear intrauterine fluid with a normal endometrium do not require treatment because this is not considered a clinically significant finding. Pediatric patients are likely to have Müllerian duct abnormalities that need surgical intervention. Postmenopausal patients who are bleeding and have a fluid collection in the uterus require evaluation of the cervix and endometrium to rule out malignancy. Those with a previous ablation that somehow spared the fundus of the uterus are a challenge and should be evaluated on an individual basis.

H

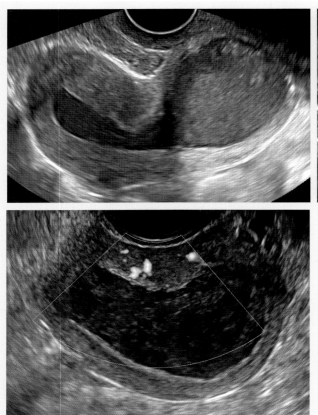

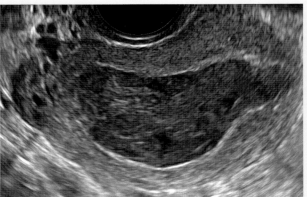

Figure H1-1   A and B, Longitudinal and transverse views of the uterus with fluid present in the cavity, including the cervix. Note that the fluid has low-level echoes, which is characteristic of unclotted blood. This was the result of an obstruction at the level of the external os. **C,** Blood flow in the myometrium but no flow within the uterine cavity.

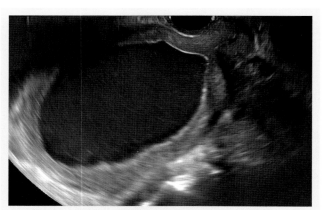

Figure H1-2   Large hematometra. Note the large fluid collection filling the uterus with a closed cervix.

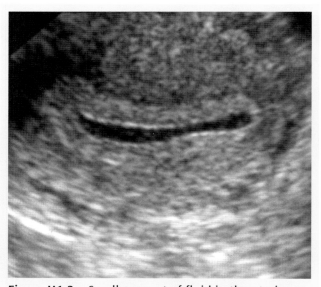

Figure H1-3   Small amount of fluid in the uterine cavity of an asymptomatic patient. With a normal-appearing endometrium, this is not considered to be clinically significant.

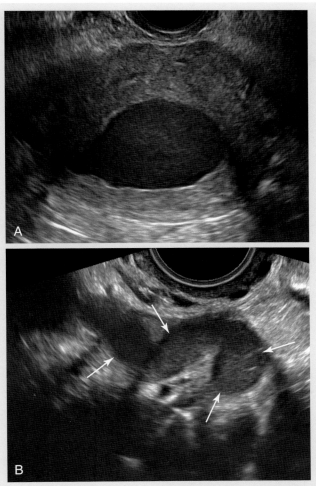

Figure H1-4   This is a patient post-endometrial ablation with pelvic pain. **A,** A transverse view through the uterine fundus showing a hematometra *(centrally).* **B,** A dilated fallopian tube full of fluid *(arrows)* with debris consistent with a hematosalpinx. The contralateral tube had the same appearance, suggesting that there is residual cycling endometrium at the uterine fundus, above the level of the ablation.

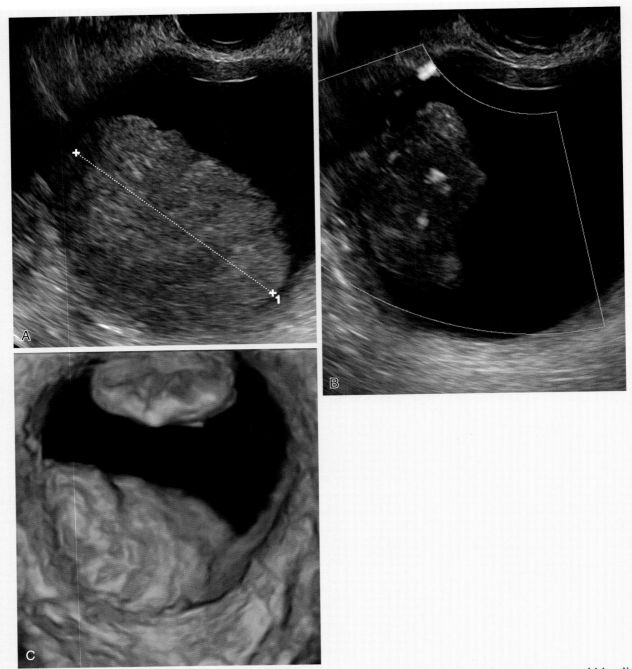

Figure H1-5   Postmenopausal patient with endometrial cancer and a 5-week history of postmenopausal bleeding. **A and B,** An endometrial mass *(calipers)* with abundant vascularity, located in the uterus and outlined by intracavitary fluid. **C,** A 3-D rendered image of the uterine cavity distended with fluid, showing two separate irregular masses in the endometrium and protruding into the cavity.

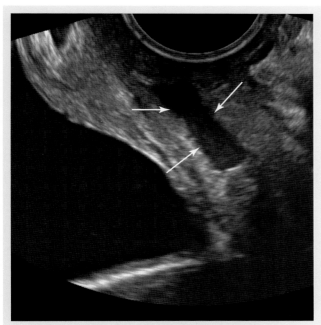

Figure H1-6 Translabial view of the vagina of a young patient with a known complex Müllerian duct abnormality. Note the obstructed hemivagina containing fluid *(arrows)*.

Suggested Reading

Goldstein SR. Postmenopausal endometrial fluid collections revisited: look at the doughnut rather than the hole. *Obstet Gynecol.* 1994;83:738-740.

Drakonaki EE, Tritou I, Pitsoulis G, Psaras K, Sfakianaki E. Hematocolpometra due to an imperforate hymen presenting with back pain: sonographic diagnosis. *J Ultrasound Med.* 2010;29:321-322.

Shaked O, Tepper R, Klein Z, Beyth Y. Hydrometrocolpos—diagnostic and therapeutic dilemmas. *J Pediatr Adolesc Gynecol.* 2008;21:317-321.

Verma SK, Baltarowich OH, Lev-Toaff AS, Mitchell DG, Verma M, Batzer F. Hematocolpos secondary to acquired vaginal scarring after radiation therapy for colorectal carcinoma. *J Ultrasound Med.* 2009;28:949-953.

Hydrosalpinx

Synonyms/Description
Fluid-filled, distended fallopian tube

Etiology
A hydrosalpinx is a dilated fallopian tube filled with fluid. A normal tube is not visible sonographically; however, when a tube becomes obstructed, it distends and fills with fluid, giving it a sausage-like appearance. Infection is a major cause of hydrosalpinx, also called pelvic inflammatory disease (PID), in which the tube fills with pus in the acute phase of the disease (pyosalpinx). In ectopic pregnancy, the tube can distend and fill with blood (hematosalpinx) and have a similar appearance to a pyosalpinx. Tubal torsion presents with acute pain and a tender, distended tube. Scarring and adhesions in the pelvis can obstruct the tubes and allow them to fill with fluid, but this is more often found in asymptomatic patients since it is not an acute process. This can also be seen in cases of severe endometriosis, or previous pelvic surgery. Rarely, tuberculosis and other infections can attack the pelvis and result in hydrosalpinx.

Ultrasound Findings
A hydrosalpinx has a typical sonographic appearance. Evaluation of the adnexa reveals a cystic, sausage-shaped, serpiginous, tubular mass. The distended tube often has a characteristic "spoke-wheel" pattern made up by the incomplete septae of the tube. The tube can become redundant and fold upon itself, giving the appearance of a multiseptate cystic mass. If the adjacent ovary is not clearly visualized, it is easy to suspect ovarian pathology. If the hydrosalpinx is the result of pelvic inflammatory disease, the tubal wall can occasionally be thick and irregular, making the correct diagnosis more difficult. In the study by Sokalska and colleagues (from the IOTA multicenter study), the sensitivity for the sonographic diagnosis of hydrosalpinx was 86%.

Hydrosalpinges are often accompanied by free pelvic fluid, especially in acute pelvic inflammatory disease or ectopic pregnancy. The presence of a solid mass within a dilated tube, along with a negative pregnancy test, may suggest fallopian tube carcinoma, although abundant vascularity would also usually be present.

Three-dimensional ultrasound is very helpful for demonstrating the course of the dilated tubes. Once a volume is obtained, the complete cast of the convoluted fallopian tube is easily seen using the inverse mode. This technique enables the practitioner to view a cast of the entire cystic tube previously hidden within the volume. The whole tube is then demonstrated, even if the tube traverses multiple planes.

Differential Diagnosis
Most hydrosalpinges are tubular fluid collections that do not conform to any single plane. Therefore with 2-D ultrasound, they can have the appearance of a multiseptate cystic mass. The "spoke-wheel" walls and a separate ovary suggest the correct diagnosis; however, too often the findings are nonspecific. Using standard 2-D sonography, the differential diagnosis includes an ovarian neoplasm or a peritoneal inclusion cyst. Volume (3-D) ultrasound with inverse mode is essential to connecting the cystic spaces into a tubal architecture if the mass is a hydrosalpinx. The patient's symptoms also play an important part in making the correct diagnosis. If a patient presents with a cystic adnexal mass and severe pain, the differential diagnosis would include pelvic inflammatory disease (signs of infection), an ectopic pregnancy (positive pregnancy test), or tubal torsion. Chronic pain or cyclic pain might indicate endometriosis. Ovarian neoplasms are often asymptomatic, but so are chronic hydrosalpinges.

A right-sided adnexal mass can be confused with an appendiceal mucocele. A dilated ureter can occasionally mimic a hydrosalpinx although the ureter typically peristalses.

Clinical Aspects and Recommendations

Most hydrosalpinges are found incidentally and are asymptomatic. Treatment, if indicated, focuses on the etiology. If the hydrosalpinx is filled with anechoic fluid, has thin walls, and the patient is asymptomatic, treatment is not typically required. Salpingectomy may be indicated for infertile patients or those with prior ectopic pregnancies desiring to conceive. Acute pelvic inflammatory disease will be treated with antibiotics, often intravenously.

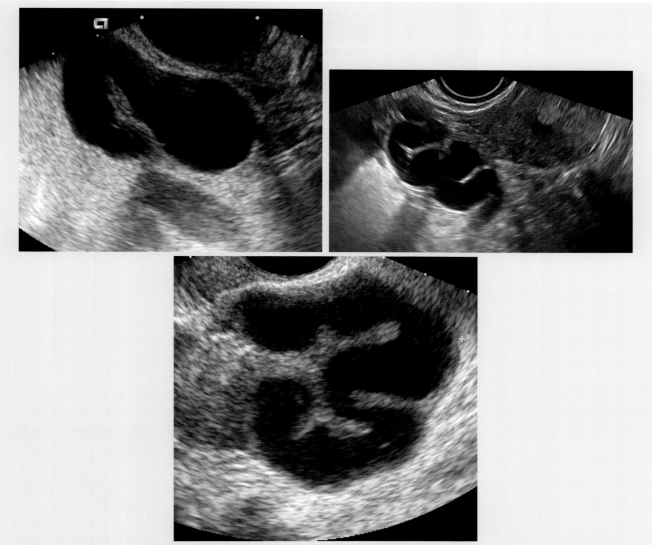

Figure H2-1　Classic sonographic appearance of a simple hydrosalpinx in three different patients. Note that the dilated tube is seen entirely in one plane, a rare finding.

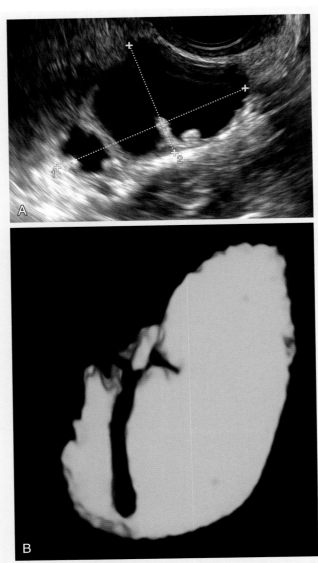

Figure H2-2 A, A 2-D sonographic image of the distal end of a hydrosalpinx, showing the typical "spoke-wheel" appearance of the incomplete septae in a dilated tube. **B,** The 3-D inverse rendering of the same tube, demonstrating the complete outer contour of the hydrosalpinx, including the bulbous blunted distal end seen in the 2-D image.

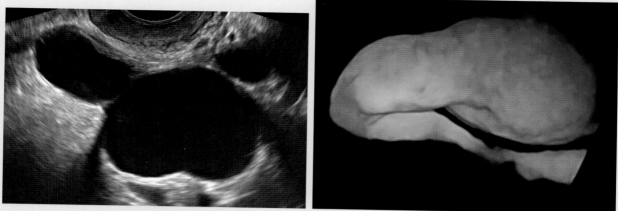

Figure H2-3   Two- and three-dimensional images of a large hydrosalpinx. The 2-D image shows several individual cysts; however, the 3-D image demonstrates that these cysts connect and represent a hydrosalpinx rather than ovarian cysts.

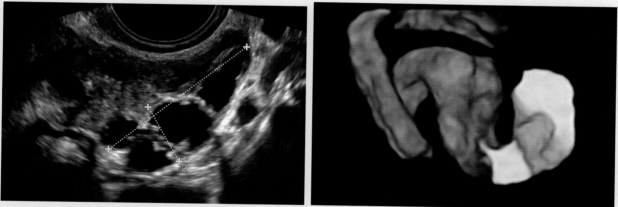

Figure H2-4   Two-dimensional image of the left adnexa showing a normal ovary with a tubular multiseptate cystic mass *(calipers)* lateral to the ovary. There are small "spoke-wheel" type incomplete septae within the cysts, but the cysts do not appear to connect to each other. The 3-D image shows that these cystic components connect into a long and narrow hydrosalpinx, confirming the diagnosis only suspected using 2-D ultrasound.

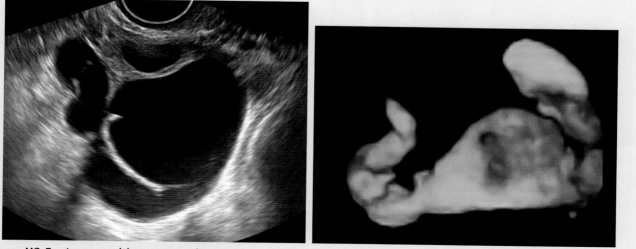

Figure H2-5   Large multiseptate cystic mass suspected to be a hydrosalpinx using 2-D ultrasound, but confirmed with 3-D inverse mode.

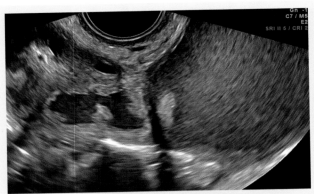

Figure H2-6   Thick-walled large hydrosalpinx in a patient with acute pelvic inflammatory disease. Note the thick and irregular wall as well as the debris and echogenic fluid in the tube consistent with a pyosalpinx.

Suggested Reading

Sokalska A, Timmerman D, Testa AC, Van Holsbeke C, Lissoni AA, Leone FPG, Jurkovic D, Valentin L. Diagnostic accuracy of transvaginal ultrasound examination for assigning a specific diagnosis to adnexal masses. *Ultrasound Obstet Gynecol.* 2009;34:462-470.

Timor-Tritsch IE, Monteagudo A, Tsymbal T. Three-dimensional ultrasound inversion rendering technique facilitates the diagnosis of hydrosalpinx. *J Clin Ultrasound.* 2010;38:372-376.

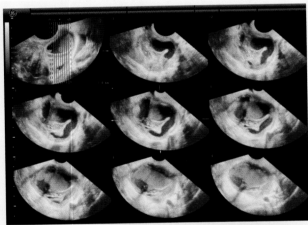

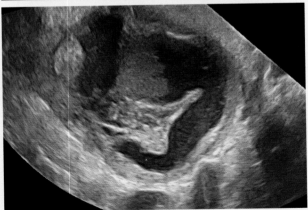

Figure H2-7   3-D images of a dilated tube containing debris in a patient with acute pelvic pain. This was proven to be torsion of the fallopian tube at surgery.

Intrauterine Device Location, Abnormal

Synonyms/Description
Mirena
ParaGard
IUD
IUCD (intrauterine contraceptive device)
LARC (long-acting reversible contraception)

Etiology
The uterus may be too small to accommodate an intrauterine device (IUD) or the IUD may not open normally because of placement or anatomic abnormalities or it may become lodged in the lower uterine segment/cervix. The IUD may become embedded in the myometrium.

Ultrasound Findings
Three-dimensional ultrasound is crucial to determining the location of an IUD. Although the shaft of the IUD is visible using 2-D ultrasound, it is often more difficult to see the relationship between the arms of the IUD and the uterine cavity, especially if the IUD did not open normally or has become bent. Sometimes the shadow of the IUD is much easier to see than the IUD itself, especially when dealing with the non–copper–containing type. The shadow of the IUD often facilitates finding the IUD by following the shadow sonographically.

Differential Diagnosis
If an IUD is in the uterus, there is most often no other diagnosis to consider. If there is a shadowing structure in the uterus, however, other etiologies can include an area of calcification from a fibroid or endometrial scarring, or a foreign body such as a laminaria. If a patient has an ultrasound immediately after an endometrial biopsy or other instrumentation of the cavity, air left in the cavity can be very bright and echogenic with a shadow, simulating an IUD. Generally, the IUDs are a typical shape that is recognizable and not usually confused with these other conditions.

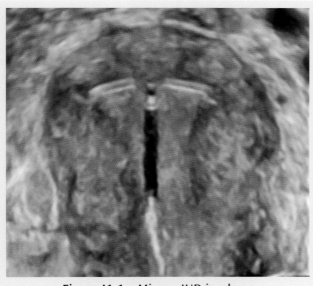

Figure I1-1   Mirena IUD in place.

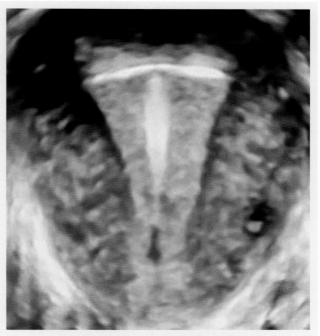

Figure I1-2   ParaGard IUD in place.

Clinical Aspects and Recommendations

An abnormally located IUD can cause pelvic pain and bleeding, although this can also be an incidental finding in an asymptomatic patient. If a patient with an IUD presents with pain or bleeding, a 3-D ultrasound should be done to evaluate the position of the device in the uterus. Malpositioned IUDs need to be removed to improve symptoms.

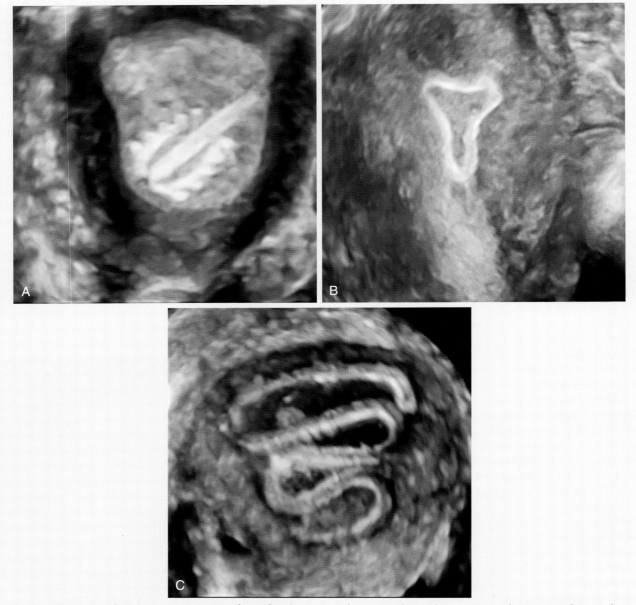

Figure I1-3   A and B, Uncommon IUDs from foreign countries. **C,** A Lippes loop IUD, no longer on the market.

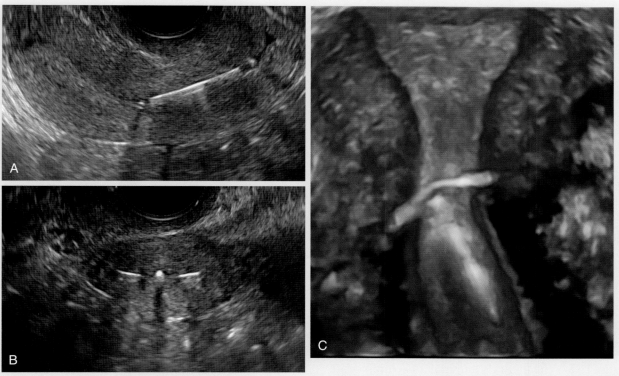

Figure I1-4 **A and B,** Longitudinal and transverse views of an IUD lodged in the cervix. **C,** The 3-D coronal view showing that the IUD is embedded in the upper cervical substance.

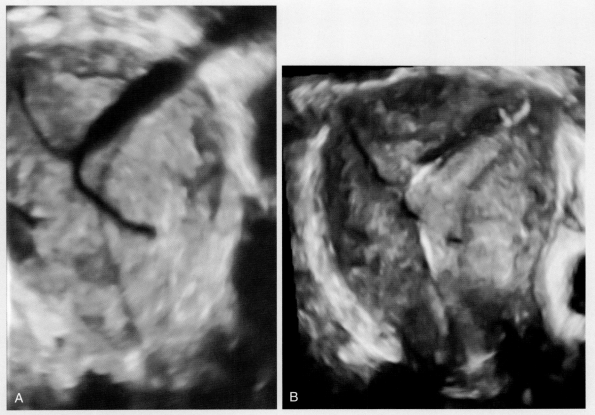

Figure I1-5 **A,** A prominent IUD shadow, upside down in the region of the left cornu. **B,** Backing the ultrasound beam in from the shadow reveals the exact position of the Mirena IUD, malpositioned across the top of the uterine cavity.

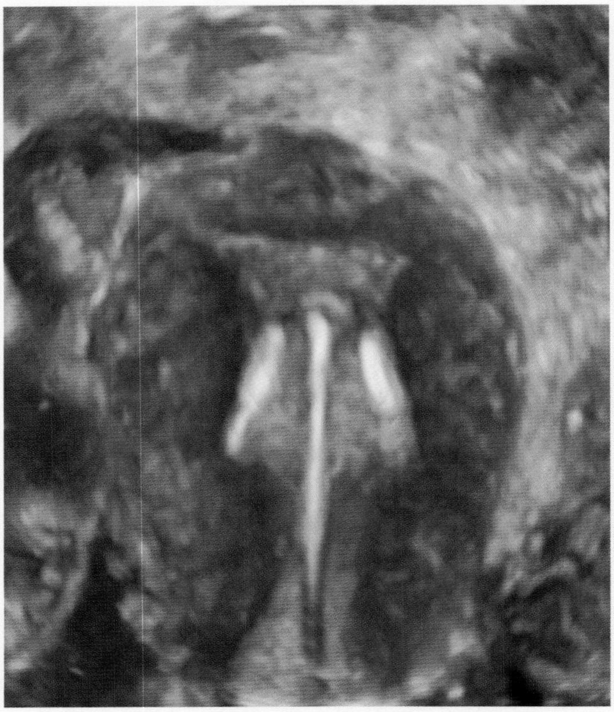

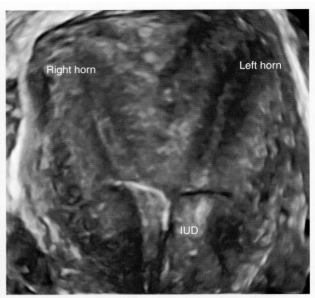

Figure I1-6   The uterus is too small to accommodate an IUD; therefore, the IUD was not able to open.

Figure I1-8   This Mirena was inserted in a septate uterus. It is lodged in the cervix as the septum blocked its placement into the uterine cavity.

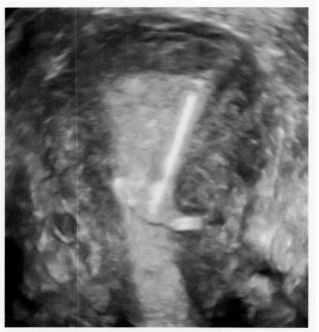

Figure I1-7   The IUD is upside down, looking like an anchor.

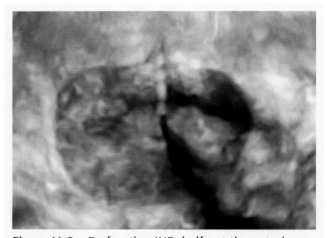

Figure I1-9   Perforating IUD, half out the anterior wall of the uterus. Note the puckering of the serosal surface of the uterus.

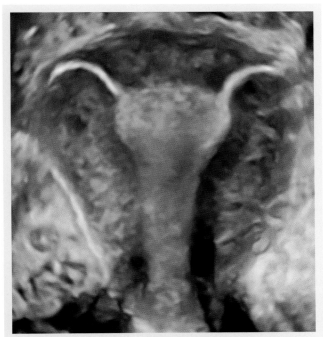

Figure I1-10　Correct placement of Essure coils in the interstitial portion of the tubes bilaterally.

Suggested Reading

Benacerraf BR, Shipp TD, Bromley B. 3D ultrasound detection of embedded intrauterine contraceptive devices—a source of pelvic pain and abnormal bleeding. *Ultrasound Obstet Gynecol.* 2009;34:110-150.

Bonilla-Musoles F, Raga F, Osborne NG, Blanes J. Control of intrauterine device insertion with three-dimensional ultrasound: is it the future? *J Clin Ultrasound.* 1996;24:263-267.

Lee A, Eppel W, Sam C, Kratochwil A, Deutinger J, Bernaschek G. Intrauterine device localization by three-dimensional transvaginal sonography. *Ultrasound Obstet Gynecol.* 1997;10:289-299.

Peri N, Graham D, Levine D. Imaging of intrauterine contraceptive devices. *J Ultrasound Med.* 2007; 26:1389-1401.

Shipp TD, Bromley B, Benacerraf BR. The width of the uterine cavity is narrower in patients with an embedded intrauterine device (IUD) compared to a normally positioned IUD. *J Ultrasound Med.* 2010;29:1453-1456.

Valsky DV, Cohen SM, Hochner-Celnikier D, Lev-Sagie A, Yagel S. The shadow of the intrauterine device. *J Ultrasound Med.* 2006;25:613-616.

Intravenous Leiomyomatosis

Synonyms/Description
Benign metastasizing leiomyoma

Etiology
This is caused by intravascular proliferation of a smooth muscle, leiomyoma-like tumor, which is noninvading locally, but grows within venous channels of the uterus and pelvis as serpiginous tubular masses. This growth can be extensive and occasionally even reach the inferior vena cava and the right atrium, causing cardiac symptoms. In one study, 56% of patients with this condition had previously had a hysterectomy for uterine fibroids.

There are two possible etiologies for this rare tumor: (1) The tumor may originate from smooth muscle in the vessel wall itself. (2) The tumor originates from a uterine leiomyoma, subsequently invading adjacent venous channels.

Ultrasound Findings
These leiomyoma-like lesions are nodular, tubular, and serpiginous solid masses in the pelvis. The intravascular location of these masses is not well seen sonographically. Color flow is typically visible within these masses. The characteristic features are tubular solid masses, often bilateral, following the course of pelvic veins.

Differential Diagnosis
Pelvic malignancies separate from the uterus and ovaries, such as sarcoma or lymphoma.

Clinical Aspects and Recommendations
This is an extremely rare condition. The disease is usually asymptomatic and will often be discovered incidentally on a chest x-ray. However, some patients will present with a cough, shortness of breath, or even chest pain. The ultimate diagnosis is based upon histologic findings of the extrauterine leiomyomas on bronchoscopic biopsy.

When the disease is asymptomatic, expectant management may be an option, although the treatment of choice for symptomatic patients is removal of the intravascular tumors as well as hysterectomy/bilateral salpingo-oophorectomy. The tumor typically contains estrogen and progesterone receptors. Thus treatment with oophorectomy and medications that induce medical menopause, such as GnRH agonists, aromatase inhibitors, or even progestins, has been shown to result in tumor regression. Usually the lesions will shrink or disappear after castration. Thus, hormone replacement therapy is usually contraindicated.

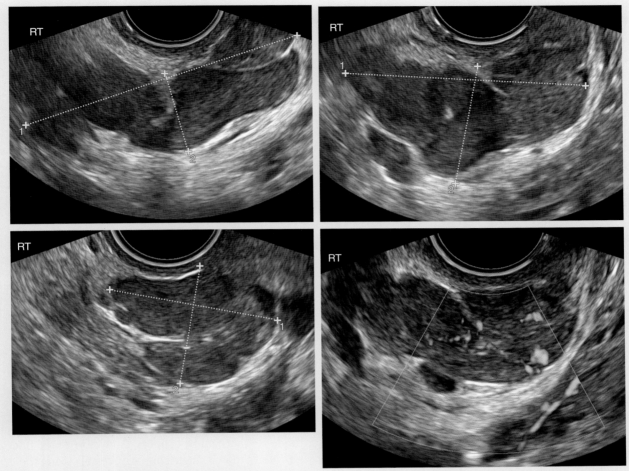

Figure I2-1　Four different views of the serpiginous and tubular solid mass in the right side of the pelvis, which was subsequently proven to be intravenous leiomyomatosis. There was abundant Doppler color flow in the mass.

Suggested Reading

Andrade LA, Torresan RZ, Sales Jr JF, Vicentini R, De Souza GA. Intravenous leiomyomatosis of the uterus. A report of three cases. *Pathol Oncol Res.* 1998;4:44-47.

Diakomanolis E, Elsheikh A, Sotiropoulou M, Voulgaris Z, Vlachos G, Loutradis D, Michalas S. Intravenous leiomyomatosis. *Arch Gynecol Obstet.* 2003;267:256-257.

Kokawa K, Yamoto M, Yata C, Mabuchi Y, Umesaki N. Postmenopausal intravenous leiomyomatosis with high levels of estradiol and estrogen receptor. *Obstet Gynecol.* 2002;100:1124-1126.

Lou YF, Shi XP, Song ZZ. Intravenous leiomyomatosis of the uterus with extension to the right heart. *Cardiovasc Ultrasound.* 2011;24(9):25.

Low G, Rouget AC, Crawley C. Intravenous leiomyomatosis with intracaval and intracardiac involvement. *AJR.* 2012;265:971-974.

Lymph Nodes, Enlarged

Synonyms/Description
Lymphadenopathy

Etiology
Lymph nodes are common sites of metastatic disease in gynecologic tumors and are an important prognostic factor in these malignancies. For example, the 5-year survival for a patient with vulvar cancer and normal nodes is 90%, compared with a patient with nodal disease, whose 5-year survival rate is 50%.

Ultrasound Findings
Normal lymph nodes (including pelvic) are typically oblong bean-shaped and small, with the transverse diameter less than or equal to 10 mm. They have a peripheral hypoechogenic band with a hyperechogenic (fatty) hilum. The vascular pattern of normal lymph nodes is characteristic, with the feeding artery and vein coursing in and out from the hilum. Lymph nodes containing tumor tend to be enlarged, with an irregular border and loss of normal sonographic architecture. They are rounded in shape rather than oblong, and their blood-flow pattern can become multifocal and disorganized.

Differential Diagnosis
Sonographically, an enlarged lymph node appears as a mass, and may be difficult to distinguish from any other solid mass in the pelvis, unless the location and pattern of blood flow suggest a lymph node. The color flow pattern of a lymph node will virtually always have a single vascular source.

Clinical Aspects and Recommendations
Ultrasound may be the initial method of detection of abnormal pelvic lymph nodes. This finding carries important prognostic and therapeutic implications and may help to stage disease in a cancer patient. PET/CT and other imaging techniques are likely to be used to further determine extent of disease and treatment.

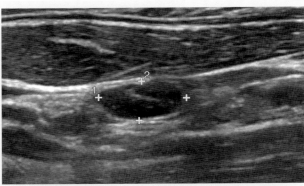

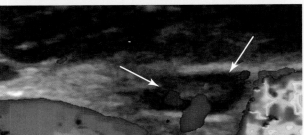

Figure L1-1 Normal lymph node. The normal lymph node is identified by calipers. Color flow to the node *(arrows)* shows a single source of vessels along the long axis of the small node.

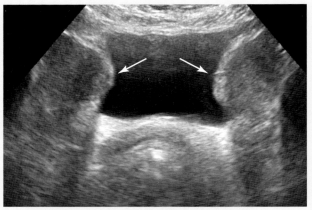

Figure L1-2 Patient with chronic lymphocytic leukemia. Transverse view of the pelvis in a patient with a full bladder showing bilateral solid masses along the pelvic side walls indenting the sides of the bladder.

L

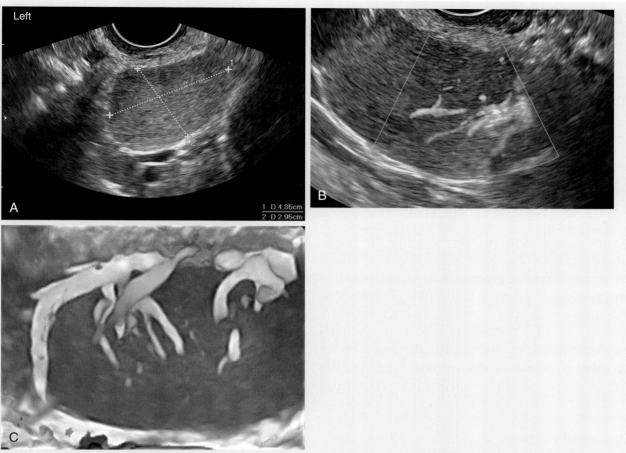

Figure L1-3 **A,** Magnified view of a left-sided mass seen transvaginally, showing a homogeneously solid mass *(calipers)*. This enlarged and abnormal node is rounded and wide, with loss of normal architecture. **B,** The same mass is interrogated with color flow Doppler, showing that the blood flow into the mass originates from one side, characteristic of a lymph node. **C,** The contralateral lymph node (seen here using 3-D color Doppler) is also enlarged with abundant color flow.

Suggested Reading

Fischerova D. Ultrasound scanning of the pelvis and abdomen for staging of gynecological tumors: a review. *Ultrasound Obstet Gynecol.* 2011;38:246-266.

Lai G, Rockall AG. Lymph node imaging in gynecologic malignancy. *Semin Ultrasound CT MRI.* 2010;31:363-376.

Gore RM, Newmark GM, Thakrar KH, Mehta UK, Berlin JW. Pelvic incidentalomas. *Cancer Imaging.* 2010;10:S15-S26.

L

Metastatic Tumor to the Ovary

Synonyms/Description
Secondary ovarian tumor
Krukenberg tumor (originating mostly from the gastrointestinal tract)

Etiology
Metastatic tumors to the ovary account for approximately 20% of ovarian malignancies. The most common primary origins for metastatic disease to the ovary include colon, stomach, breast, and the genitourinary tract, and less commonly, lymphoma and leukemia. Krukenberg tumor is a specific term, characteristically used to describe metastatic colon or stomach adenocarcinoma to the ovary, although breast and other sites may be the primary. Spread of the primary tumor to the ovaries may occur from direct seeding or, more likely, via lymphatics.

Ultrasound Findings
Metastases to the ovaries are bilateral in 60% to 80% of cases, especially when the primary malignancy originates from the stomach, colon, rectum, or breast.

Krukenberg tumors are bilateral in more than 70% of cases. They are typically large masses containing solid and cystic components. Frequently the mass is multiloculated with a multitude of small cystic compartments intermixed with solid areas, giving a frothy sonographic appearance. More than 50% of Krukenberg tumors have associated ascites, especially when there is bilateral disease. It is not uncommon to have the Krukenberg tumor be the initial symptom or finding, while the primary has not yet been discovered. Reportedly, up to 7% of ovarian lesions presenting as primary ovarian malignancies are actually metastatic in origin.

Metastatic tumors from nongastrointestinal origin tend to be more solid and smaller than those from a gastrointestinal origin.

Differential Diagnosis
Metastatic tumors to the ovary can have a similar appearance to primary ovarian malignancies. Both can be complex cystic and solid masses associated with ascites. The bubbly or frothy appearance of the mass, often large and bilateral, is a feature that should raise suspicion for metastatic adenocarcinoma of the gastrointestinal tract rather than a primary ovarian cancer.

Often the smaller unilateral masses are nonspecific-appearing and cannot be accurately diagnosed as a primary or secondary malignancy. Abundant color flow is usually present in these malignant tumors, whether they are primary or secondary. The presence of abundant color flow would make a benign etiology unlikely.

Clinical Aspects and Recommendations
The prognosis of secondary ovarian tumors is typically poor; patients with gastric cancer metastatic to the ovaries usually succumb to the disease within 1 year. The treatment for malignancies that have metastasized to the ovary varies according to the primary tumor. Management may include a combination of oncologic and surgical approaches.

M

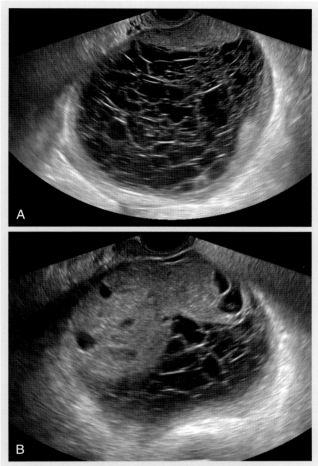

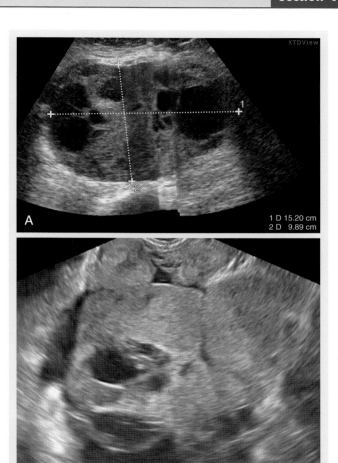

Figure M1-1 A and B, Metastatic colon cancer to the ovary—Krukenberg tumor. Note the multiple tiny cystic areas and septations, giving a frothy appearance. **B** shows that part of the mass is solid.

Figure M1-2 A and B, Adenocarcinoma of the stomach metastatic to the ovary—Krukenberg tumor. Note the large size of the tumor with multiple small cystic areas within a solid matrix.

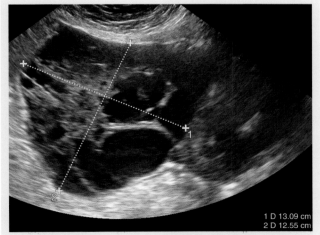

Figure M1-3 Colon cancer metastatic to the ovary. Note the large size of the mass, which is typical.

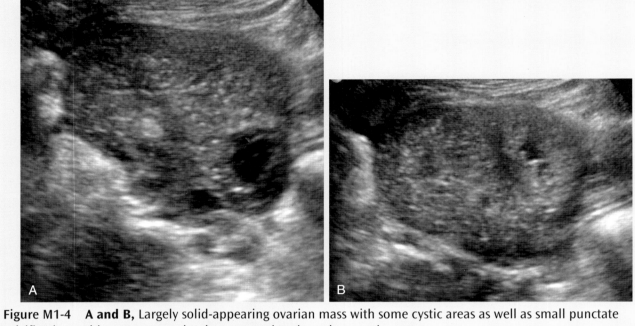

Figure M1-4   A and B, Largely solid-appearing ovarian mass with some cystic areas as well as small punctate calcifications. This tumor proved to be metastatic colon adenocarcinoma.

M

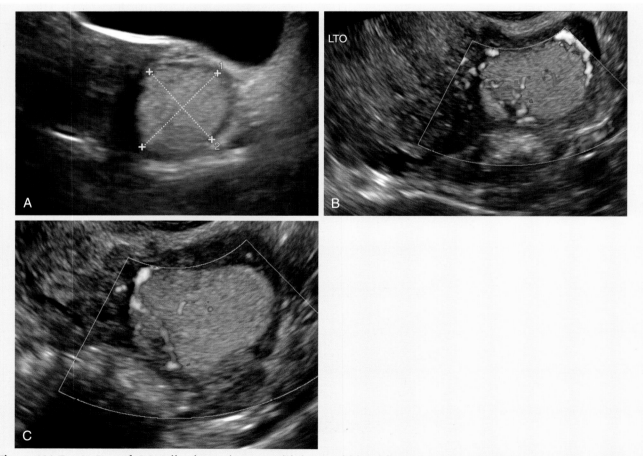

Figure M1-5   A, B, and C Small echogenic mass with internal blood flow shown on Doppler examination (**B and C**). This proved to be an adenocarcinoma originating from the appendix and metastatic to the ovary, first presenting as an adnexal mass.

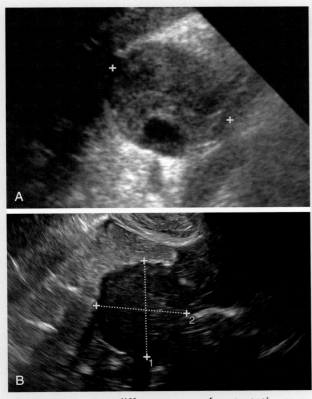

Figure M1-6 Two different cases of metastatic breast cancer to the ovary. Both are small tumors that are largely solid, although **A** shows a small cystic portion.

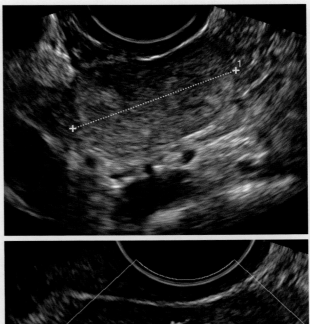

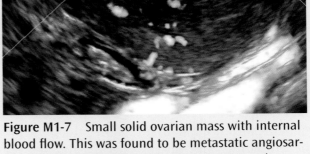

Figure M1-7 Small solid ovarian mass with internal blood flow. This was found to be metastatic angiosarcoma of the ovary at surgery. The appearance is nonspecific sonographically, although suspected to be a malignancy.

Suggested Reading

Guzel AB, Gulec UK, Paydas S, Khatib G, Gumurdulu D, Vardar MA, Altintas A. Preoperative evaluation, clinical characteristics, and prognostic factors of nongenital metastatic ovarian tumors: review of 48 patients. *Eur J Gynaecol Oncol.* 2012;33(5): 493-497.

Jain V, Guptay K, Kudvay R, Rodrigues GS. A case of ovarian metastasis of gall bladder carcinoma simulating primary ovarian neoplasm: diagnostic pitfalls and review of literature. *Int J Gynecol Cancer.* 2006;16(suppl. 1):319-321.

Koyama T, Mikami Y, Saga T, Tamai K, Togashi K. Secondary ovarian tumors: spectrum of CT and MR features with pathologic correlation. *Abdom Imaging.* 2007;32:784-795.

Loke TKL, Lo SS, Chan CS. Case report: Krukenberg tumours arising from a primary duodenojejunal adenocarcinoma. *Clin Radiol.* 1997;52:154-155.

Yada-Hashimoto N, Yamamoto T, Kamiura S, Seino H, Ohira H, Sawai K, Kimura T, Saji F. Metastatic ovarian tumors: a review of 64 cases. *Gynecol Oncol.* 2003;89:314-317.

M

Mucinous Cystadenoma

Synonyms/Description
One of the epithelial-stromal tumors containing mucoid material

Etiology
Most mucinous cystadenomas are benign tumors, although 20% can be borderline (low malignant potential) or malignant. Benign mucinous cystadenomas represent 20% to 25% of all benign ovarian tumors and occur mostly during the third to fifth decades. These mucinous tumors are comprised most often of the mucin-producing cell type similar to a cell type that lines the intestinal tract, although a minority of the tumors have endocervical-like mucin-producing cells. Some tumors may contain both cell types.

Borderline mucinous cystadenomas are of low malignant potential and carry a 5-year survival prognosis of 95%. The less common borderline the endocervical type has a worse prognosis and higher recurrence rate than the intestinal type. For the borderline and invasive neoplasms, see elsewhere in this book.

Ultrasound Findings
Mucinous cystadenomas are multilocular in 50% of cases, with solid components or papillary projections in 40% of borderline and malignant cases. The fluid inside the cystic area typically contains low-level echoes much like an endometrioma; however, when interrogated with Doppler, the echoes stream compared with those in endometriomas, which usually do not. The different compartments of the cystic mass may differ as to the texture of the echoes within, likely secondary to different cell types within a single tumor. When internal nodules with blood flow are present, the possibility of a borderline or invasive malignancy must be considered. Typically, borderline malignancies have fewer nodules and less blood flow within them compared with invasive tumors, although this is a very subjective finding.

Differential Diagnosis
The differential diagnosis includes any complex cystic mass of the adnexa. These diagnoses are numerous and include serous cystadenoma, cystadenofibroma, endometrioma, peritoneal inclusion cyst, degenerating fibroid, complex hydrosalpinx, and so on. It may not be possible to arrive at a specific diagnosis sonographically when faced with a multiseptate cystic mass; however, the characteristic finding to consider in a mucinous cystadenoma is the presence of low-level echoes, much like an endometrioma but with multiple septations. Often a patient with endometriosis will be symptomatic and may have other sites of endometriotic implants that would differentiate it from a single asymptomatic mass such as a cystadenoma. If a separate ovary can be found, the differential might include non-ovarian diagnoses such as hydrosalpinx or peritoneal inclusion cyst.

Clinical Aspects and Recommendations
Like any adnexal mass, mucinous cystadenomas may present with pelvic pain, especially during activities such as intercourse, exercise, or defecation. However, most commonly they are asymptomatic and are appreciated on routine bimanual pelvic examination or incidentally found at the time of pelvic imaging for virtually any indication. Benign mucinous ovarian neoplasms can become extremely large and thus come to surgical exploration. When they are multilocular, they may raise suspicion for malignancy. Increasingly, however, a minimally invasive approach using laparoscopic surgery is favored over laparotomy, especially to preserve ovarian function when the mass is considered benign. Although less common, when unilocular and small, these

M

masses can be treated expectantly. Tumor markers such as CA125 are elevated in less than 50% of malignant neoplasms, and thus would not be expected to be extremely helpful in such cases. If conservative management is undertaken, follow-up sonographic surveillance at periodic intervals is appropriate.

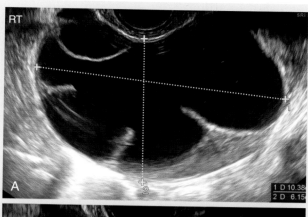

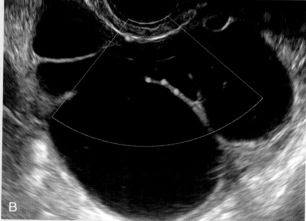

Figure M2-3   A and B, Multiseptate mucinous cystadenoma with fine septations containing color flow but no nodularity.

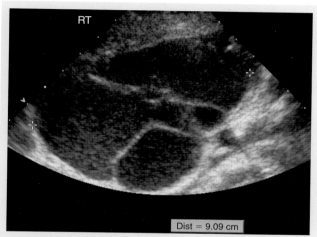

Figure M2-1   Typical mucinous cystadenoma. Note the diffuse low-level echoes with multiple septations.

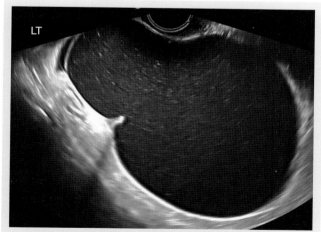

Figure M2-2   Unilocular cystadenoma with typical but somewhat coarse low-level echoes caused by the mucinous secretions.

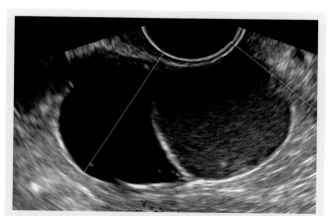

Figure M2-4   Mucinous cystadenoma with low-level echoes in one portion, typical of this type of tumor, in which there are different echo textures in each compartment.

M

Suggested Reading

Caspi B, Hagay Z, Appelman Z. Variable echogenicity as a sonographic sign in the preoperative diagnosis of ovarian mucinous tumors. *J Ultrasound Med.* 2006;25:1583-1585.

Fruscella E, Testa AC, Ferrandina G, De Smet F, Van Holsbeke C, Scambia G, Zannoni GF, Ludovisi M, Achten R, Amant F, Vergote I, Timmerman D. Ultrasound features of different histopathological subtypes of borderline ovarian tumors. *Ultrasound Obstet Gynecol.* 2005;26:644-650.

Hart WR. Mucinous tumors of the ovary: a review. *In J Gynecol Pathol.* 2005;24:4-25.

M

Müllerian Duct Anomalies

Synonyms/Description
Congenital uterine anomalies

Etiology
Congenital anomalies of uterine shape occur in 3% to 4% of all women. The prevalence in women with infertility and early miscarriage is up to 10%, and as high as 25% in those with midtrimester pregnancy losses. Patients with uterine shape abnormalities have an increased incidence of congenital renal anomalies such as unilateral renal agenesis. The American Society for Reproductive Medicine has developed the following classification of uterine anomalies.

Class I: Agenesis of the Uterus, Cervix, and/or Upper Vagina
Includes women with Mayer-Rokitansky-Küster-Hauser syndrome (incidence 1/5000). Patients with this condition are born with no uterus, cervix, or upper vagina.

Class II: Unicornuate Uterus (20% of Uterine Anomalies)
This anomaly results from a lack of or incomplete development of one of the two Müllerian tubercles. This gives rise to only one complete horn of the uterus with either total absence or hypoplasia of the contralateral horn (rudimentary horn). In 35% of cases, the unicornuate uterus is isolated, but most are associated with variable development of a contralateral rudimentary uterine horn. Thirty-three percent of women with a unicornuate uterus have a noncavitary rudimentary horn (without endometrium), whereas 32% have a rudimentary horn with endometrium present. This rudimentary horn may or may not communicate with the "normal" hemiuterus.

Unicornuate uteri are associated with an early pregnancy loss rate of 41% to 62%, especially when a rudimentary horn is present. They are also associated with preterm delivery.

Class III: Didelphic Uterus (5% of Uterine Anomalies)
These patients have a complete lack of fusion of the bilateral Müllerian ducts, resulting in two totally separate uterine horns, each with its own endometrial cavity and cervix. The vagina also contains a septum in 75% of cases. Uterine didelphys is associated with spontaneous miscarriage rates of 32% to 52% and premature birth rates of 20% to 45%.

Class IV: Bicornuate Uterus (10% of Uterine Anomalies)
Incomplete fusion of the two Müllerian ducts leads to a concave dip in the serosal surface of the uterine fundus as well as a division of the endometrial cavity into two horns that connect near the cervix. Bicornuate uteri are associated with spontaneous abortion rates of 28% to 35% and premature birth rates of 14% to 23%.

Class V: Septate Uterus (55% of Uterine Anomalies)
When there is absence of normal resorption of the uterine septum after the two Müllerian ducts have fused, the uterine cavity will be septate. The septum may be complete or partial (more common), but the serosal surface of the uterus remains normal. A uterine septum is associated with spontaneous abortion rates ranging from 26% to 94% and premature birth rates ranging from 9% to 33%.

Class VI: Arcuate Uterus
This is considered a normal variant. With a normal serosal surface, these uteri have a slight indentation of the fundal portion of the uterine cavity that measures less than 1 cm in depth.

M

Ultrasound Findings

Before 3-D ultrasound, 2-D ultrasound was the first imaging modality to suspect a Müllerian duct anomaly; however, MRI was needed to display the coronal view of the uterine cavity to make the correct diagnosis. Although the hysterosalpingogram accurately depicts the shape of the uterine cavity, it provides no information about the outer contour of the uterus. A hysterosalpingogram cannot distinguish between a septate and a bicornuate uterus.

Currently, 3-D ultrasound can easily provide a reconstructed coronal view of the uterus, demonstrating both the shape of the endometrial cavity and the outer serosal/myometrial contour of the uterus. MRI is no longer necessary to diagnose the vast majority of uterine malformations. The accuracy of both 3-D ultrasound and MRI for diagnosing specific uterine malformations is 90% to 95%.

Once a 3-D image of the coronal view of the uterine cavity is obtained, the anatomy of the uterus can be observed easily. The uterus is septate if the septum extends 10 mm or more into the cavity from the midcornual line and the serosal surface is normal. A septum that is shallow and extends less than 10 mm caudally defines an arcuate uterus. A bicornuate uterus has a serosal indentation extending 10 mm or more caudally from the normal serosal surface, thus creating two horns. The bicornuate uterus also has an obligatory septum or partial septum, called a subseptum. Patients with Müllerian duct anomalies may have two cervices (bicollis), which are visible using 3-D reconstruction of the cervix. A uterine didelphys has two completely separate uterine horns that are located at opposite sides of the pelvis. These two horns are typically hard to image simultaneously because of their distance from each other.

Differential Diagnosis

The 3-D coronal view of the uterus is very accurate, and there is usually no differential diagnosis when the image is adequate. It is sometimes difficult to decide whether the uterus is arcuate or partially septate, and admittedly the criteria are rather arbitrary, probably with some overlap clinically. The same is true for the borderline bicornuate uterus in which the serosal dip may not quite reach 10 mm.

The unicornuate uterus may have a bizarre-looking rudimentary horn, which can mimic a solid mass such as a fibroid. In such cases, the presence of the unicornuate anatomy of the uterus should suggest the correct diagnosis of a rudimentary horn.

Clinical Aspects and Recommendations

All types of uterine anomalies are associated with renal anomalies. Women with a unicornuate uterus have the highest prevalence of renal anomalies, occurring in approximately 40%. Although all uterine anomalies are associated with a multitude of reproductive complications, the only type amenable to definitive treatment is the septate uterus. Hysteroscopic resection of a uterine septum is a relatively successful procedure in expert hands. Removal of a uterine septum is not always necessary and should be based on the patient's reproductive history and desires, the size of the septum, and consultation with experts in this area. Because all forms of uterine anomalies are associated with certain types of obstetric complications, these patients require differing degrees of surveillance during pregnancy. Consultation or management by maternal-fetal medicine experts should be considered.

M

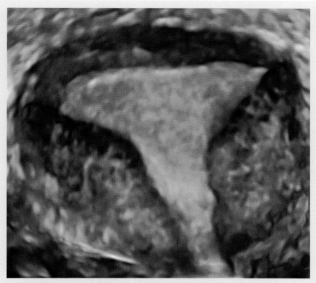

Figure M3-1 The normal uterine cavity seen using the 3-D coronal view. Note the triangular shape of the uterine cavity and the rounded outer myometrial wall or serosal surface of the uterus.

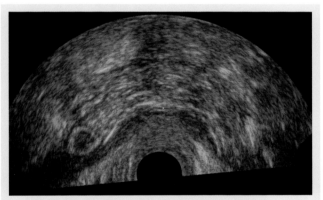

Figure M3-2 Mayer-Rokitansky-Küster-Hauser syndrome. Note the absence of the uterus and cervix in the pelvis. The vaginal probe could only be inserted part of the way into the vagina. The rest of the vagina is not developed.

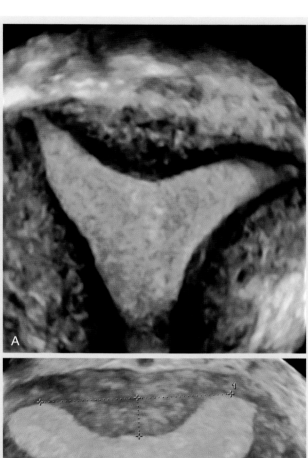

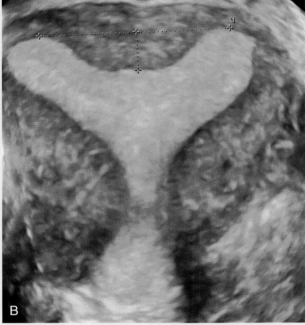

Figure M3-3 **A and B,** Two different patients with arcuate uteri. **B** shows the proper way to measure the depth of the myometrial indentation. If the measurement is 10 mm or more, then it is a septum. The measurement was less than 10 mm, indicating an arcuate uterus.

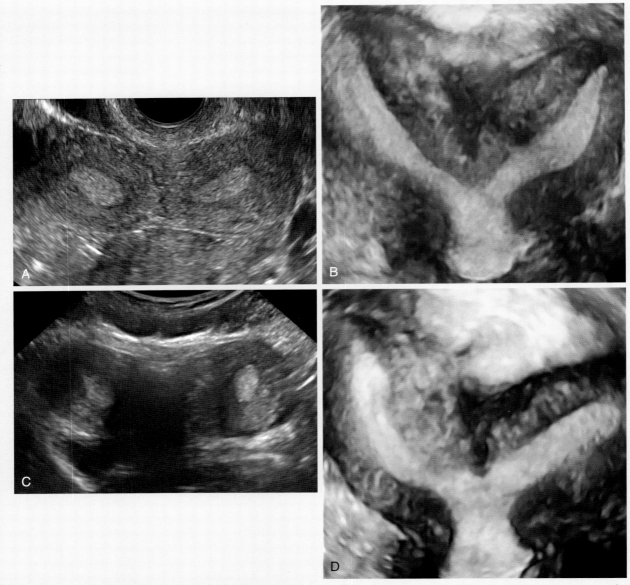

Figure M3-4 Bicornuate uterus seen in 2-D and 3-D in two different patients. The 2-D image is a transverse view through the fundus of the uterus, showing two islands of endometrium and indicating a Müllerian anomaly. The 3-D image shows the typical bicornuate uterus with a deep indentation at the fundus, dividing the uterus into two distinct horns. These horns merge in the lower uterine segment. Figures **A** and **B** are one patient and **C** and **D** are another.

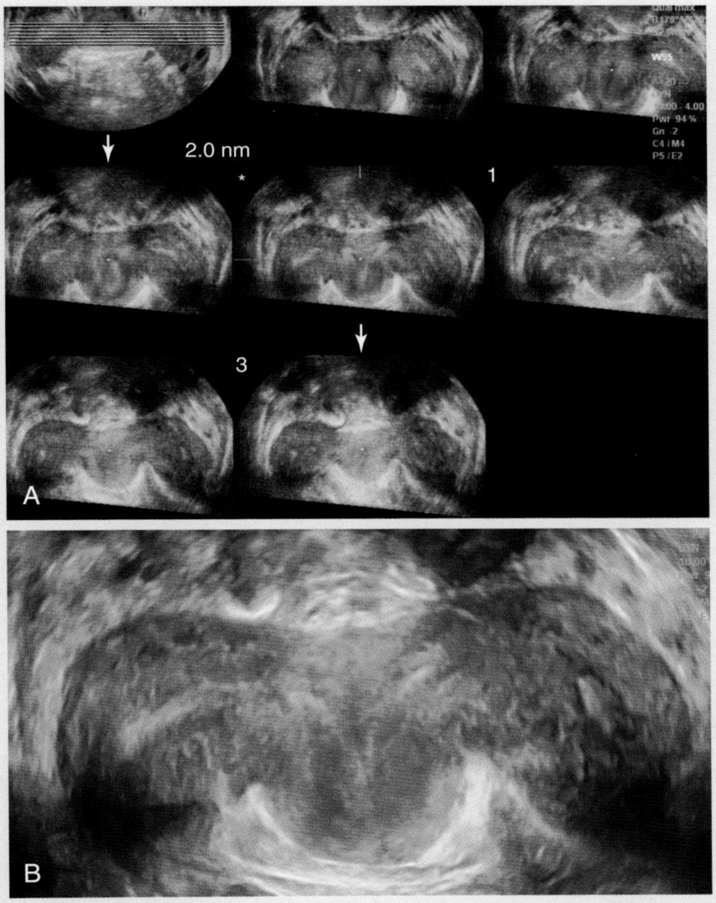

Figure M3-5   A and B, Uterus didelphys. Note that the two uterine horns are widely separated and take on the appearance of floppy rabbit ears on this 3-D coronal view.

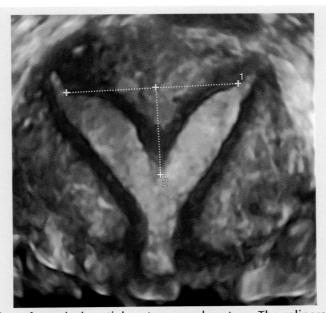

Figure M3-6   3-D coronal view of a typical partial septum or subseptum. The calipers demonstrate the method of measuring the depth of the septum.

M

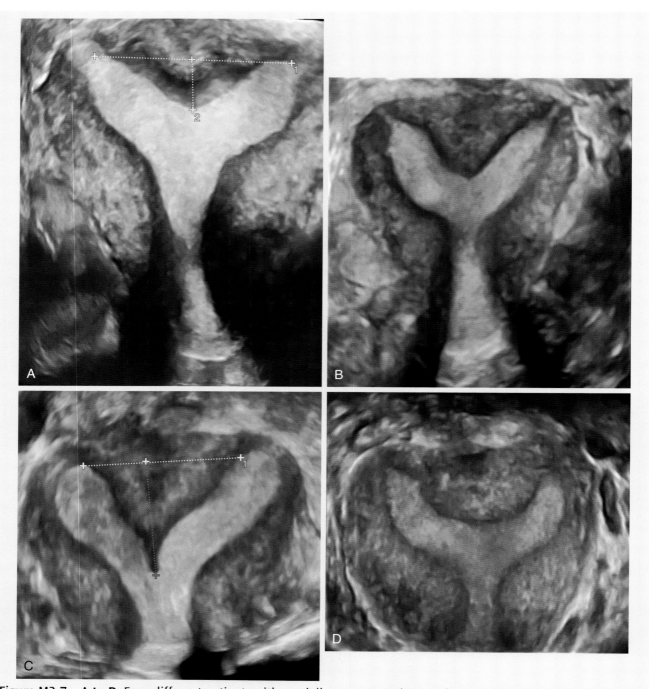

Figure M3-7 **A to D,** Four different patients with partially septate uteri. Note the very different widths and depths of the septae when comparing the appearance of these uteri. The smallest septum (**A**) measured 12 mm and has an appearance similar to the arcuate uterus in Figure M3-3.

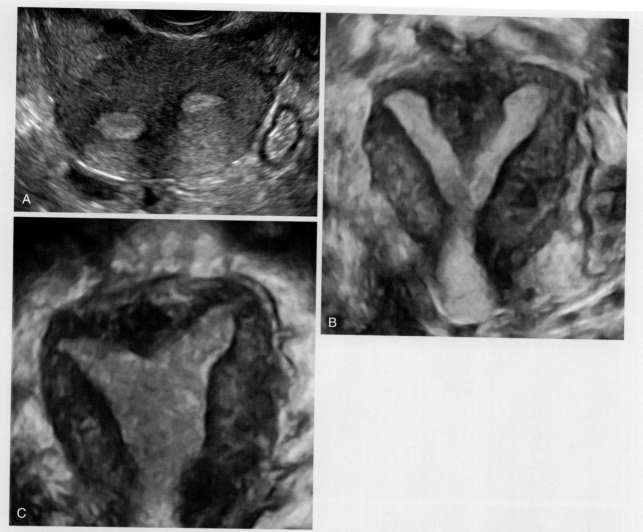

Figure M3-8   A partially septate or subseptate uterus. **A** is a 2-D transverse view, showing the typical two islands of endometrium consistent with a Müllerian anomaly. **B** shows the preoperative 3-D coronal view of the partial septum. **C** shows the postoperative result of the septal excision.

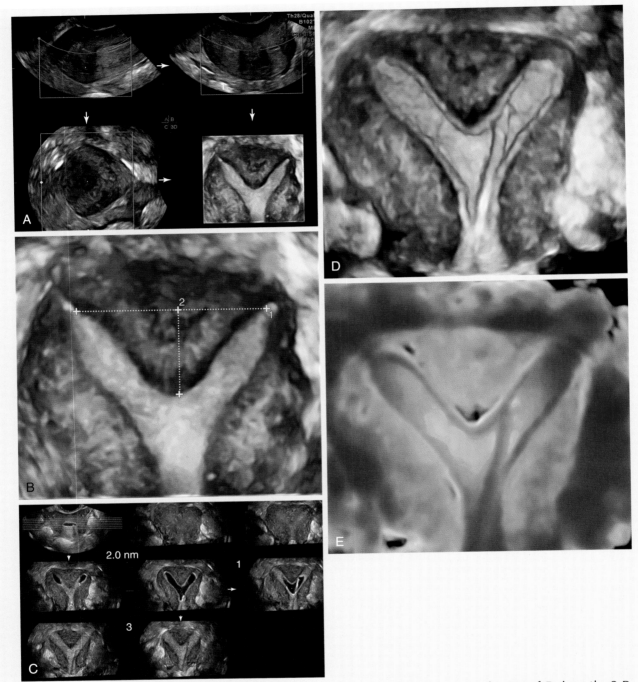

Figure M3-9   Partially septate/subseptate uterus seen using 3-D and sonohysterography. **A and B** show the 3-D volume displaying the partial septum. **C to E** show the sonohysterogram images of the same septum (**C** is a parallel tomographic cut through the uterus). Note that the catheter is visible inside the left endometrial cavity.

M

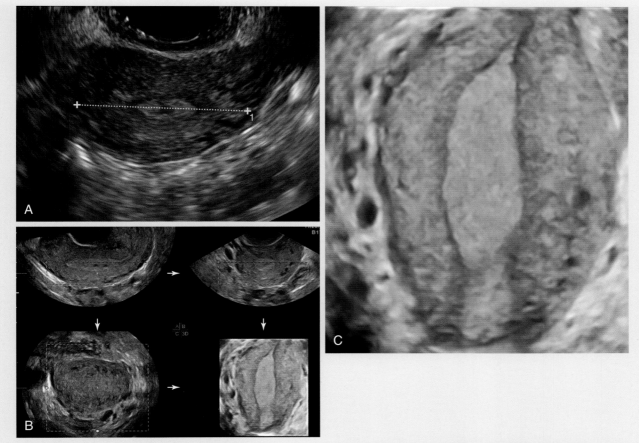

Figure M3-10 Unicornuate uterus. **A** shows a unicornuate uterus seen with 2-D ultrasound. The anomaly is very hard to detect on this view. **B and C** show the single uterine horn using 3-D ultrasound. The 3-D rendered coronal view makes the anomaly obvious.

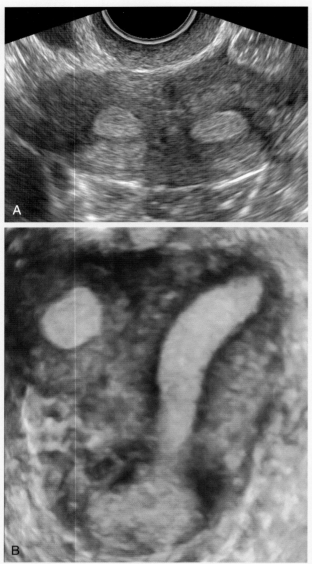

Figure M3-11   A and B, Unicornuate uterus with a noncommunicating rudimentary horn. **A,** The 2-D image suggests a septate uterus; however, the 3-D coronal view **(B)** demonstrates the rudimentary horn with an island of endometrium, which does not connect with the rest of the cavity.

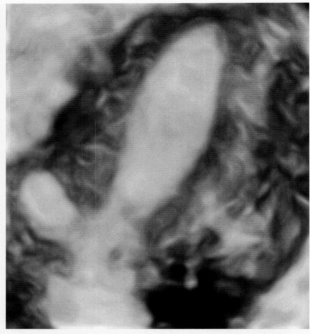

Figure M3-12   Unicornuate uterus with a small rudimentary horn. Note that the rudimentary horn contains a small cavity that connects to the rest of the uterus but is tiny.

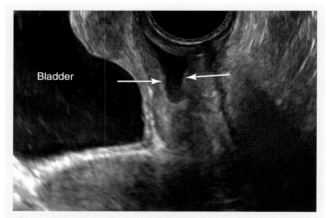

Figure M3-13   Obstructed hemivagina. This patient had a didelphic uterus, and there was a fluid collection in the vaginal region. This is a view from the perineum looking up into the vagina. Note the fluid collection *(arrows)*, indicating an obstructed hemivagina.

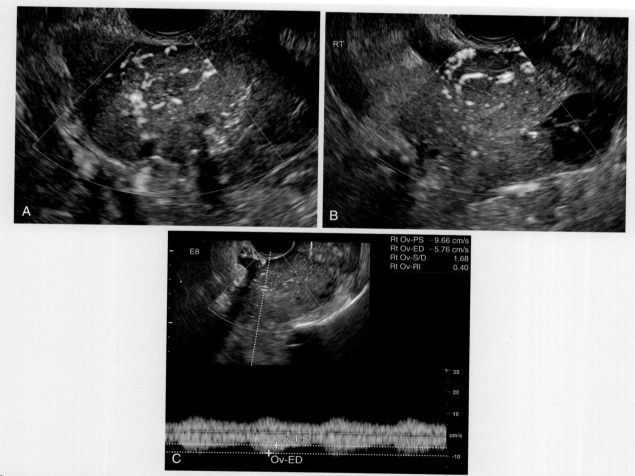

Figure O2-1   Seven-centimeter ovarian cancer. Transvaginal view of the solid-appearing mass with abundant vascularity with irregular, jagged vessels.

Figure O2-2   A to C, Ovarian cancer. Nine-centimeter ovarian cancer showing small cystic areas within a largely solid mass with extensive vascularity. **C** shows the low resistive index of 0.4 using spectral Doppler. This abundant diastolic flow is frequently seen in malignant tumors; however, the mere presence of disorganized blood vessels in the center of the mass is the most important Doppler finding.

O

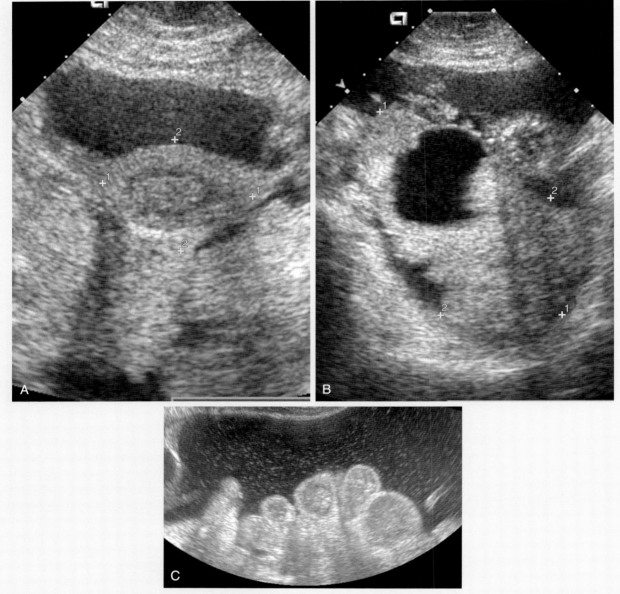

Figure O2-3   Advanced ovarian cancer. **A** shows a large amount of ascites anterior to the uterus *(calipers)* on a transverse view of the pelvis. **B** shows the large complex irregular mass *(calipers)*, which was the ovarian tumor. Note the surrounding ascites. **C** shows the extensive ascites surrounding bowel loops, higher up in the abdomen.

O

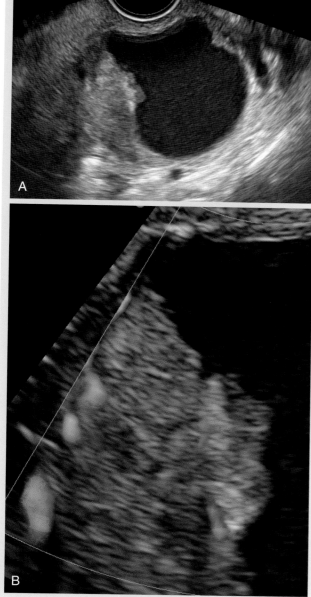

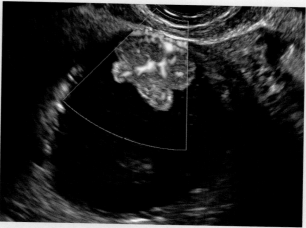

Figure O2-5 Serous cystadenocarcinoma in a pregnant patient who presented for a routine 9-week obstetric scan. Note the typical deranged and irregular branching vascularity within the nodule.

Figure O2-4 Clear cell carcinoma. **A** shows a largely cystic tumor with areas of nodularity that are often associated with endometriosis. **B** shows that the solid nodules contain blood flow, which is a characteristic of malignancy.

O

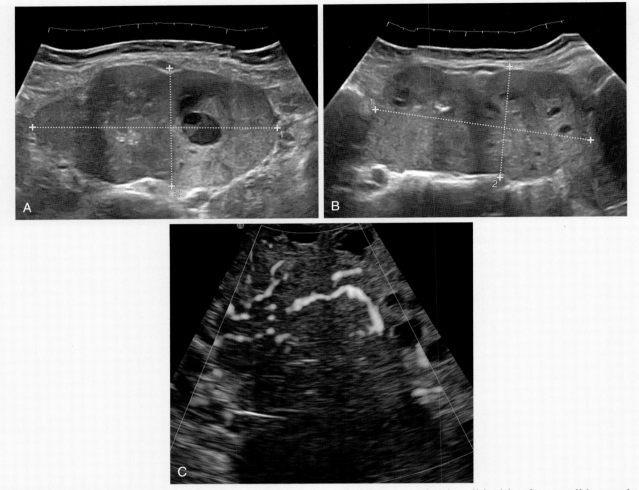

Figure O2-6   A and B, Very large serous cystadenocarcinoma, almost completely solid with a few small internal cysts. **C** shows the intense vascularity with typical disorganized tumor vessels.

O

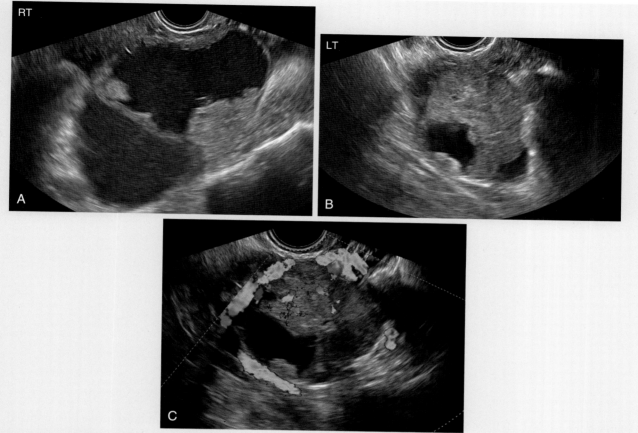

Figure O2-7 Bilateral papillary serous cystadenocarcinoma. **A** shows the right-sided lesion, which is predominantly cystic with several solid areas and a thick septum. **B and C,** The left-sided lesion is mostly solid with a small cystic component.

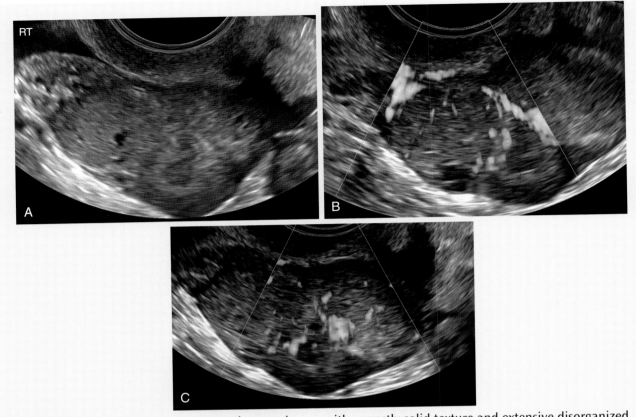

Figure O2-8   A to C, Typical serous cystadenocarcinoma with a mostly solid texture and extensive disorganized vascularity.

0

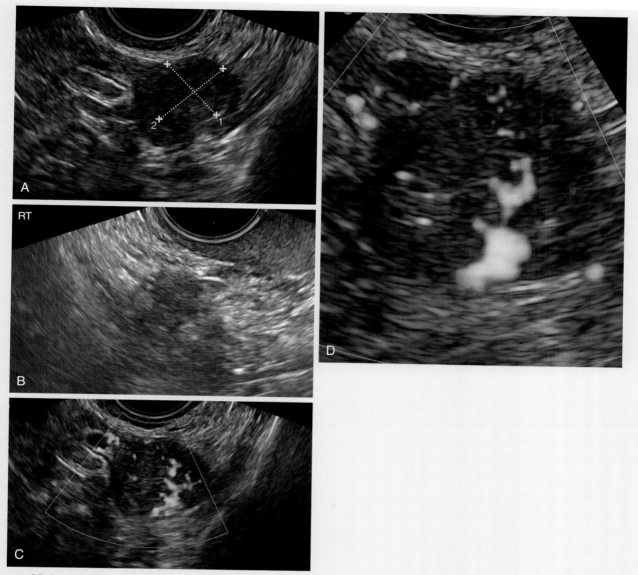

Figure O2-9 Stage 1 ovarian cancer in a 73-year-old patient. **A** shows an enlarged left ovary with a subtle 1.5-cm solid mass *(calipers)*. **B** shows the normal (small) right ovary for comparison. **C and D** show the abundant blood flow to the small tumor. Typically it is difficult to demonstrate blood vessels within a normal postmenopausal ovary, making the flow pattern in the left ovary abnormal.

O

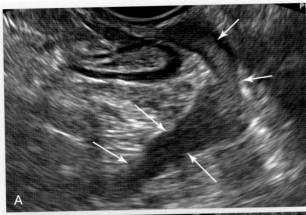
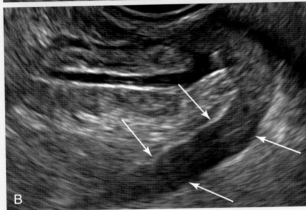

Figure O2-10   A and B, Primary extraovarian peritoneal carcinoma. Arrows show the linear solid mass coating the lateral side wall of the pelvis and peritoneal cavity.

Videos

Video 1 on ovarian cancer (epithelial) is available online.

Suggested Reading

Alcázar JL, Rodriguez D. Three-dimensional power Doppler vascular sonographic sampling for predicting ovarian cancer in cystic-solid and solid vascularized masses. *J Ultrasound Med.* 2009;28:275-281.

Ameye L, Valentin L, Testa AC, Van Holsbeke C, Domali E, Van Huffel S, Vergote I, Bourne T, Timmerman D. A scoring system to differentiate malignant from benign masses in specific ultrasound-based subgroups of adnexal tumors. *Ultrasound Obstet Gynecol.* 2009;33:92-101.

Campbell S. Ovarian cancer: role of ultrasound in preoperative diagnosis and population screening. *Ultrasound Obstet Gynecol.* 2012;40:245-254.

Kaijser J, Bourne T, Valentin L, Sayasneh A, Van Holsbeke C, Vergote I, Testa AC, Franchi D, Van Calster B, Timmerman D. Improving strategies for diagnosing ovarian cancer: a summary of the International Ovarian Tumor Analysis (IOTA) studies. *Ultrasound Obstet Gynecol.* 2013;41:9-20.

Sharma A, Apostolidou S, Burnell M, Campbell S, Habib M, Gentry-Maharaj A, Amso N, Seif MW, Fletcher G, Singh N, Benjamin E, Brunell C, Turner G, Rangar R, Godfrey K, Oram D, Herod J, Williamson K, Jenkins H, Mould T, Woolas R, Murdoch J, Dobbs S, Leeson S, Cruickshank D, Fourkala EO, Ryan A, Parmar M, Jacobs I, Menon U. Risk of epithelial ovarian cancer in asymptomatic women with ultrasound-detected ovarian masses: a prospective cohort study within the UK collaborative trial of ovarian cancer screening (UKCTOCS). *Ultrasound Obstet Gynecol.* 2012;40:338-344.

Timmerman D, Ameye L, Fischerova D, Epstein E, Melis GB, Guerriero S, Van Holsbeke C, Savelli L, Fruscio R, Lissoni AA, Testa AC, Veldman J, Vergote I, Van Huffel S, Bourne T, Valentin L. Simple ultrasound rules to distinguish between benign and malignant adnexal masses before surgery: prospective validation by IOTA group. *BMJ.* 2010;341:c6839.

Timmerman D, Valentin L, Bourne TH, Collins WP, Verrelst H, Vergote I. Terms, definitions and measurements to describe the sonographic features of adnexal tumors: a consensus opinion from the International Ovarian Tumor Analysis (IOTA) Group. *Ultrasound Obstet Gynecol.* 2000;16:500-505.

Vang R, Shih EM, Kurman RJ. Fallopian tube precursors of ovarian low- and high-grade serous neoplasms. *Histopathology.* 2013;62:44-58.

Ovarian/Tubal Torsion

Synonyms/Description
Adnexal torsion

Etiology
Torsion is defined as the twisting by at least one complete turn of the adnexa, ovary, or (rarely) the tube only around the infundibulo-pelvic and tubo-ovarian ligament, resulting in ischemia. It occurs more frequently on the right side (70%), perhaps because of a longer tubo-ovarian ligament on the right. Approximately 15% of ovarian torsions occur in children. An increase in weight of the adnexa is the primary risk factor for torsion, particularly with dermoid cysts and other mobile ovarian masses. Ovarian cancer or endometriomas seldom cause torsion because of lack of mobility of these lesions. The incidence of ovarian torsion increases during pregnancy, and ovarian stimulation is an additional risk factor.

Up to 26% of cases of torsion occur in patients who have an apparently normal adnexa; therefore a leading ovarian mass is not always present.

Paratubal cysts weighing down the tube can cause isolated torsion of the tube, although this is rare compared with ovarian torsion. Occasionally a torsed fallopian tube is associated with a hydrosalpinx.

Ultrasound Findings
An adnexal mass in a patient with pain should prompt consideration of adnexal torsion as a diagnosis. The typical appearance of a torsed ovary is a large, edematous ovary with multiple, small, peripherally placed follicles and heterogeneous texture of the ovarian stroma. The ovary may be very large and tender during the scan. If color Doppler reveals no blood flow in the ovary, then the diagnosis of torsion can be made confidently. The presence of flow, however, cannot be used to rule out adnexal torsion. Blood flow to the ovary may be intermittent or diminished because venous flow may be obliterated, but arterial flow may still be present. The ovary also has a dual blood supply, which may confound the Doppler findings. Doppler interrogation of the twisted vascular pedicle may reveal a spiral appearance of the vessels, referred to as the "whirlpool" sign. A positive whirlpool sign has a high positive predictive value for diagnosing torsion and should be part of the evaluation in a symptomatic patient.

The detection rate of torsion is reportedly only between 46% and 74%, likely because of the nonspecific findings associated with this entity and lack of expertise in recognizing them.

Isolated tubal torsion is rare, and it typically mimics a hydrosalpinx such that differentiation between an uncomplicated hydrosalpinx and tubal torsion is difficult. The whirlpool sign can be very helpful when considering tubal torsion.

Differential Diagnosis
A patient with ovarian or tubal torsion typically presents with fairly acute, worsening pelvic pain. This is often, although not always, accompanied by nausea, vomiting, and fever. The clinical differential diagnosis includes appendicitis, ureteral calculi, diverticulitis, colitis, ectopic pregnancy, pelvic inflammatory disease, and ruptured or hemorrhagic ovarian cyst. The presence of an adnexal mass narrows the differential diagnosis to a tubo-ovarian abscess (TOA), an ectopic pregnancy, a hemorrhagic cyst, or torsion. Color Doppler may help because a TOA is associated with excessive blood flow caused by inflammation, and an ectopic pregnancy can be excluded by a negative pregnancy test. An inflamed appendix can occasionally be confused with an adnexal mass; however, the tubular configuration of the appendix should help to exclude ovarian torsion, and a normal ovary usually can be visualized transvaginally.

O

Clinical Aspects and Recommendations

Adnexal or ovarian torsion is a gynecologic surgical emergency, and quick diagnosis is essential. If the diagnosis is made early and normal blood flow is restored, the adnexa may be saved. If the diagnosis is missed or delayed, ischemia will eventually result in necrosis of the ovary and/or fallopian tube. The longer surgical treatment is delayed, the more severe the sequelae because of increasing release of cytokines, which can result in sepsis and more severe systemic sequelae.

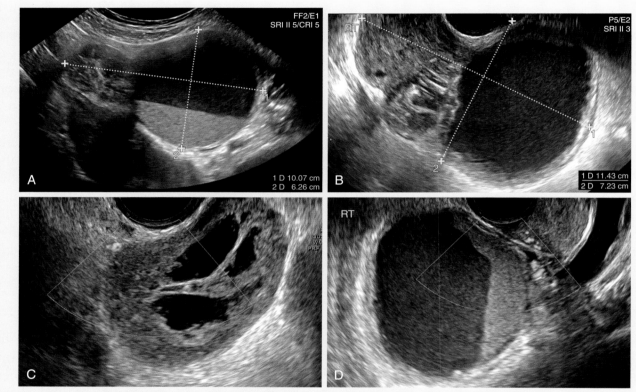

Figure O3-1   Adolescent girl with a 1-month history of pelvic pain. Endometriosis was the diagnosis initially given before referral. **A** shows a large pelvic mass seen anterior to the uterus on a transabdominal scan *(calipers)*. **B to D** show various transvaginal views of the mass, which has both cystic and solid components. Note that there is complete absence of blood flow to the ovary. The diagnosis of torsion was made based on these findings, and the patient was taken to surgery.

0

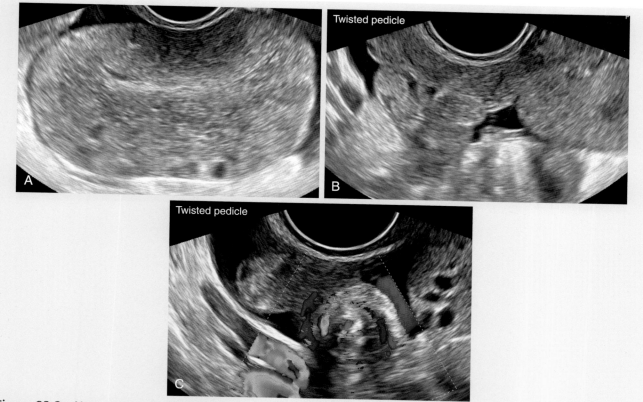

Figure O3-2   Young, reproductive-age woman with a 2-day history of acute pelvic pain. Local diagnosis of ovarian tumor was made. **A** shows the huge edematous ovary with a few peripheral follicles. **B** shows the edematous twisted pedicle. **C** shows color Doppler of the whirlpool sign of the twisted pedicle.

0

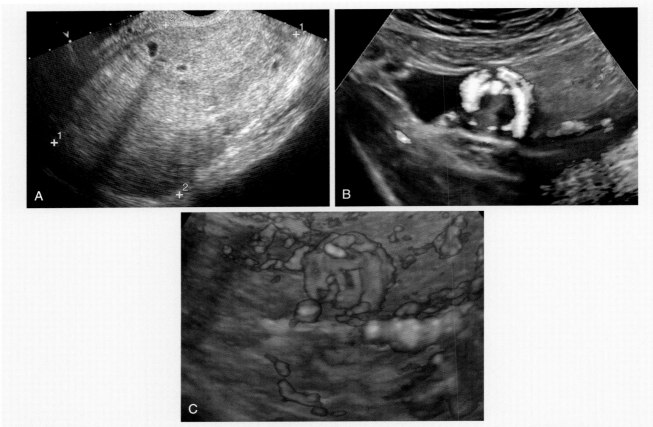

Figure O3-3 **A,** Transvaginal view of a huge pelvic mass with no blood flow. Note the severely edematous ovary with a few peripheral follicles. **B and C** show the twisted vascular pedicle or positive whirlpool sign in 2-D and 3-D.

0

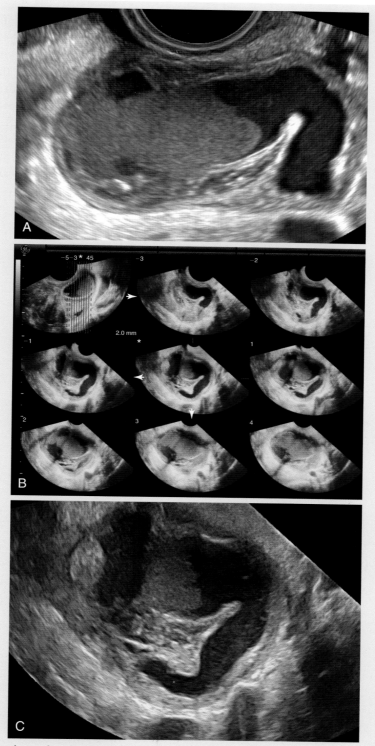

Figure O3-4 Torsed fallopian tube. **A** shows a hydrosalpinx with a very thickened wall and debris within the tube. **B and C** show 3-D of the tube, demonstrating the complex-appearing fluid and debris within the swollen tube. The diagnosis of torsion was made at surgery.

O

Videos

Video 1 on ovarian/tubal torsion is available online.

Suggested Reading

Boukaidi SA, Delotte J, Steyaert H, Valla JS, Sattonet C, Bouaziz J, Bongain A. Thirteen cases of isolated tubal torsions associated with hydrosalpinx in children and adolescents, proposal for conservative management: retrospective review and literature survey. *J Pediatr Surg.* 2011;46:1425-1431.

Huchon C, Fauconnier A. Adnexal torsion: a literature review. *Eur J Obstet Gynecol Reprod Biol.* 2010:1508-1512.

Servaes S, Zurakowski D, Laufer MR, Feins N, Chow JS. Sonographic findings of ovarian torsion in children. *Pediatr Radiol.* 2007;37(5):446-451.

Valsky DV, Esh-Broder E, Cohen SM, Lipschuetz M, Yagel S. Added value of the gray-scale whirlpool sign in the diagnosis of adnexal torsion. *Ultrasound Obstet Gynecol.* 2010;36:630-634.

Vijayaraghavan SB, Senthil S. Isolated torsion of the fallopian tube: the sonographic whirlpool sign. *Ultrasound Med.* 2009;28:657-662.

Wilkinson C, Sanderson A. Adnexal torsion—a multimodality imaging review. *Clin Radiol.* 2012;67:476-483.

0

Ovarian Vein Thrombosis

Synonyms/Description
Septic pelvic thrombophlebitis (SPT)

Etiology
Ovarian vein thrombosis is a rare but potentially severe postpartum complication, occurring 80% to 90% of the time on the right side, and with a reported incidence of 1:600 to 1:2000 deliveries. Ovarian vein thrombosis can also occur in the immediate postoperative period after pelvic surgery or in conjunction with pelvic infection or thrombophilias such as factor V Leiden mutation. Spontaneous ovarian vein thrombosis without any of these predisposing conditions is exceedingly rare.

The ovarian veins are located in the retroperitoneum, anterior to the psoas muscle. The right ovarian vein is longer than the left, and it drains into the inferior vena cava below the right renal vein. The left drains into the left renal vein.

Ultrasound Findings
Ovarian vein thrombosis appears as a hypoechoic tubular mass cephalad to the ovary. Color Doppler typically shows an absence of flow within the mass.

The sensitivity, specificity, and accuracy of ultrasound with Doppler are reportedly 55.6%, 41.2%, and 46.2%, respectively. The sonographic evaluation is often limited by overlying bowel gas because the ovarian vein is a retroperitoneal structure; therefore CT with contrast is often used to make a more definitive diagnosis.

Differential Diagnosis
A tubular painful mass in the right lower quadrant can mimic appendicitis. The ultrasound findings may be similar, although the appendix is typically located more anteriorly in the abdomen than is the ovarian vein, which is more dorsal. Doppler is also helpful in differentiating these two diagnoses, as abundant color flow is seen in the walls of the appendix and ovarian vein thrombosis has little flow. Other possible but less likely diagnoses when dealing with a painful lower quadrant mass, especially if left-sided, include ovarian torsion, broad ligament fibroid, hydrosalpinx, and pelvic inflammatory disease. The presence of a separate ovary, location of the mass, and color Doppler pattern are very helpful to arrive at the correct diagnosis.

Clinical Aspects and Recommendations
Ovarian vein thrombosis should be considered in postpartum patients who present with abdominal or flank pain (right more frequently) and with fever, typically spiking, that is unresponsive to broad-spectrum antibiotics. These symptoms often mimic appendicitis, tubo-ovarian abscess, ovarian torsion, or broad ligament hematoma. Treatment is usually medical and may include parenteral broad-spectrum antibiotics with the addition of anticoagulant therapy.

If untreated, ovarian vein thrombosis can lead to inferior vena cava and renal vein thrombosis, pulmonary thromboembolism, and sepsis.

O

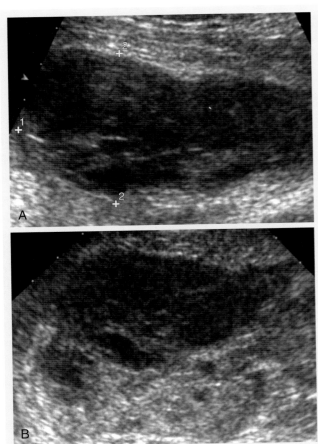

Figure O4-1   A and B, Longitudinal and transverse views of the right ovarian vein showing a hypoechoic mass with internal strandy echoes consistent with internal organizing clot. No blood flow was identified using Doppler color flow.

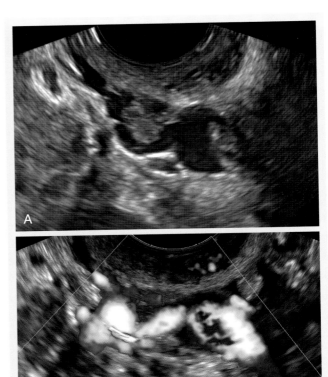

Figure O4-2   A and B, Longitudinal view of the right external iliac containing multiple clots incidentally noted on a gynecologic scan. **B** shows color Doppler of the vein in the same projection, showing defects within the color consistent with clot. The thrombosis was confirmed with contrast CT, and the patient was anticoagulated.

Suggested Reading

Bilgin M, Sevket O, Yildiz S, Sharifov R, Kocakoc E. Imaging of postpartum ovarian vein thrombosis. *Case Rep Obstet Gynecol.* 2012;2012:134603.

Dewdney SB, Benn T, Rimel BJ, Gao F, Saad N, Vedantham S, Mutch DG, Zighelboim I. Inferior vena cava filter placement in the gynecologic oncology patient: a 15-year institutional experience. *Gynecol Oncol.* 2011;121:344-346.

Sharma P, Abdi S. Ovarian vein thrombosis. *Clin Radiol.* 2012;67:893-898.

Stafford M, Fleming T, Khalil A. Idiopathic ovarian vein thrombosis: a rare cause of pelvic pain—case report and review of literature. *Aust N Z J Obstet Gynaecol.* 2010;50:299-301.

O

Paratubal or Paraovarian Cysts

Synonyms/Description
Adnexal cyst, mesothelial or paramesonephric cyst

Etiology
Paratubal and paraovarian cysts arise from the broad ligament. They constitute 10% of adnexal masses. They are usually benign but may rarely (reportedly 2%) contain malignant or borderline elements.

Etiologies for paratubal cysts include mesosalpingeal cysts, hydatid cysts of Morgagni, and paratubal subserosal cysts arising from Müllerian duct remnants, as opposed to paraovarian cysts, which arise from mesonephric tubules (Wolffian duct) and are mesothelial in origin.

Ultrasound Findings
Paratubal and paraovarian cysts are typically unilocular thin-walled adnexal cysts that are separate from the ovaries. Paratubal cysts are usually farther removed from the ovaries than paraovarian cysts, which are usually adjacent to the ovary. These cysts can (rarely) cause tubal or adnexal torsion or undergo hemorrhage or rupture, resulting in severe pelvic pain. Occasionally paratubal or paraovarian cysts can have septations, nodularities, and excrescences, suggesting a malignancy (occurs in 2% of such cysts).

Differential Diagnosis
The presence of a thin-walled, clear adnexal cyst separate from the ovary is considered to be a paratubal or paraovarian cyst. The differential diagnosis may include a hydrosalpinx (although the tubal wall is thicker than that of a cyst) or a peritoneal inclusion cyst (usually contains multiple septations and takes on the shape of the adjacent peritoneal surface). It is important to identify the ovary separately; otherwise, an ovarian etiology is possible, especially if the cyst is not simple and unilocular.

Clinical Aspects and Recommendations
Most paratubal or paraovarian cysts are incidental findings and asymptomatic. When patients present with pelvic pain, the cysts may have undergone hemorrhage, torsion, or rupture. If the cyst has thick septations, an irregular wall, or nodularity, a neoplasm (cystadenoma, cystadenocarcinoma, or borderline tumor) should be considered.

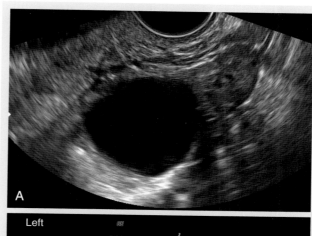
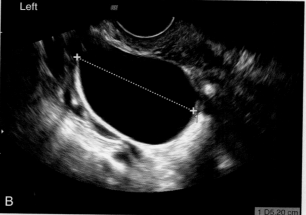

Figure P1-1   A and B, Two views of a simple paraovarian cyst

P

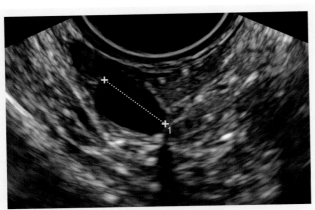

Figure P1-2 Typical unilocular paratubal cyst. Note that there is no ovarian tissue visible. The ovary was totally separate from the cyst.

Suggested Reading

Barloon TJ, Brown BP, Abu-Yousef MM, Warnock NG. Paraovarian and paratubal cysts: preoperative diagnosis using transabdominal and transvaginal sonography. *J Clin Ultrasound.* 1996;24:117-122.

Kim JS, Woo SK, Suh SJ, Morettin LB. Sonographic diagnosis of paraovarian cysts: value of detecting a separate ipsilateral ovary. *Am J Roentgenol.* 1995;164:1441-1444.

Kiseli M, Caglar GS, Cengiz SD, Karadag D, Yilmaz MB. Clinical diagnosis and complications of paratubal cysts: review of the literature and report of uncommon presentations. *Arch Gynecol Obstet.* 2012;285:1563-1569.

Stein AL, Koonings PP, Schlaerth JB, Grimes DA, d'Ablaing 3rd G. Relative frequency of malignant parovarian tumors: should parovarian tumors be aspirated? *Obstet Gynecol.* 1990;75:1029-1031.

Terek MC, Sahin C, Yeniel AO, Ergenoglu M, Zekioglu O. Paratubal borderline tumor diagnosed in the adolescent period: a case report and review of the literature. *J Pediatr Adolesc Gynecol.* 2011;24:e115-e116.

P

Pelvic Congestion Syndrome

Synonyms/Description
Varicose veins of the pelvis

Etiology
Although the etiology of pelvic congestion syndrome is unclear, it appears that gross dilatation, valve incompetence, and reflux of the ovarian veins may be causal. Anatomic and/or hormonal factors may lead to insufficiency of the ovarian and/or internal iliac veins, resulting in peri-ovarian pelvic varicosities. Such tubo-ovarian varicoceles may be the female equivalent of testicular varicoceles.

Ultrasound Findings
The ultrasound diagnosis is based on a subjective impression of excessive venous channels in a patient with dull and chronic pelvic pain made worse when standing. CT scans have also been used to detect these varicosities, but an ultrasound diagnosis is usually sufficient. The objective criteria include dilated ovarian veins greater than 4 mm in diameter, dilated and tortuous arcuate veins communicating with pelvic varicose veins, and retrograde venous flow, particularly in the left ovarian vein.

Differential Diagnosis
The diagnosis of pelvic venous congestion is suggested after all other causes of pelvic pain have been excluded. Endometriosis is a common cause of chronic pelvic pain that should be investigated before implicating venous congestion as a final diagnosis. Furthermore, there are patients with large pelvic veins who have no pain at all and others who barely make the subjective criteria for this disorder but who complain of debilitating pain. Certainly once a patient has been investigated for other causes of pelvic pain, large, dilated, tortuous pelvic varicosities with sluggish and occasional retrograde flow do suggest the diagnosis of pelvic venous congestion syndrome.

Clinical Aspects and Recommendations
Clinically, pelvic congestion syndrome is characterized by pelvic pain of at least 6 months duration. It often manifests during or after a pregnancy and worsens with subsequent pregnancies. Such pain can be variable in its severity, but it is usually described as a dull ache or heaviness. It increases premenstrually and is worsened with prolonged standing, postural changes, walking, or activities that can increase intra-abdominal pressure. Occasionally it is worsened after intercourse. Classically it is unilateral and greater on the left side in most patients. It is virtually unheard of in menopausal women, thus implicating the hormone estrogen in part of the pathogenesis.

There is no standard approach to treatment of pelvic congestion syndrome. Ovarian cycle suppression with combination contraceptives, GnRH agonists, or high-dose progestational agents has been employed. In the most severe cases refractory to medical management, embolization of ovarian veins can be performed. Rarely, hysterectomy and bilateral salpingo-oophorectomy can be viewed as a last resort.

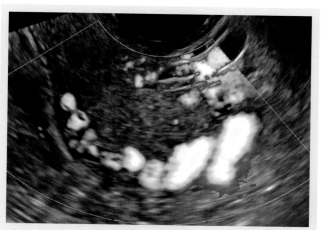

Figure P2-1 Color flow Doppler image showing excessive and large veins around the uterus in a patient with characteristic dull but chronic pelvic pain.

P

Suggested Reading

Beard RW, Reginald PW, Wadsworth J. Clinical features of women with chronic lower abdominal pain and pelvic congestion. *Br J Obstet Gynecol.* 1988;95:153.

Hobbs JT. The pelvic congestion syndrome. *Br J Hosp Med.* 1990;43:200.

Ignacio EA, Dua R, Sarin S, Harper AS, Yim D, Mathur V, Venbrux AC. Pelvic congestion syndrome: diagnosis and treatment. *Semin Intervent Radiol.* 2008;25:361-368.

Tu FF, Hahn D, Steege JF. Pelvic congestion syndrome-associated pelvic pain: a systematic review of diagnosis and management. *Obstet Gynecol Surv.* 2010;65:332-340.

P

Pelvic Kidney

Synonyms/Description
Ectopic location of kidney—normal variant

Etiology
The incidence of pelvic kidney is reported as being between 1 in 2200 and 1 in 3000. The normal human kidney migrates to the renal fossa from a pelvic location early in embryonic development, typically before the 10th week of gestation. The congenital failure of this migration results in a pelvic kidney. Although a pelvic kidney is defined as a normal variant, it is associated with Müllerian duct anomalies such as uterine malformation (see Müllerian Duct Anomalies). Pelvic kidney is the most common type of renal ectopia and is typically clinically asymptomatic. However, ectopically located kidneys are at increased risk of urinary tract infection, stone formation, and trauma.

Ultrasound Findings
Pelvic kidneys that have a normal reniform appearance can easily be recognized as an ectopic kidney. It is important to check the corresponding renal fossa to confirm the absence of the kidney in its normal location before diagnosing a pelvic kidney. If there are cysts or fluid collections associated with the pelvic kidney, the correct diagnosis may be more challenging, and it is crucial to consider the diagnosis of ectopic kidney with hydronephrosis and hydroureter. The patient may also have an associated uterine anomaly, so a transvaginal gynecologic ultrasound should be included as part of the evaluation.

Differential Diagnosis
An abnormal-appearing pelvic kidney may result in misdiagnosis when there is hydronephrosis, large cystic structures, or stones. Ureteropelvic junction (UPJ) obstruction has been reported in 22% to 37% of ectopic kidneys. A cystic or hydronephrotic kidney may be mistaken for an adnexal cystic mass such as an ovarian neoplasm or hydrosalpinx (in the case of a dilated ureter). Ectopic kidneys are associated with Müllerian duct anomalies, which may further confuse the sonographic appearance of the other pelvic organs.

Clinical Aspects and Recommendations
Pelvic kidneys are most often incidental and not clinically significant; however, they are associated with Müllerian duct anomalies, which can cause significant reproductive, mostly obstetric, complications. Therefore when an ectopic kidney is identified in a patient of reproductive age, sonographic evaluation of the reproductive tract, preferably 3-D, must be documented.

Occasionally, ectopic kidneys can be diseased and related to lower abdominal pain if there are renal stones, hydronephrosis, or cysts or pyelonephritis. Rarely, renal masses such as malignancies have been identified in pelvic kidneys.

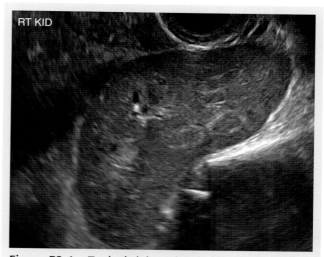

Figure P3-1 Typical right pelvic kidney seen transvaginally, adjacent to the vaginal probe. It is important not to mistake this structure for a solid pelvic mass.

P

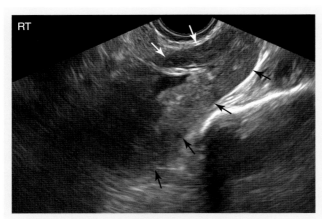

Figure P3-2 Right pelvic kidney *(arrows)* with a common malrotation, which resulted in mild hydronephrosis.

Suggested Reading

Cinman NM, Okeke Z, Smith AD. Pelvic kidney: associated diseases and treatment. *J Endourol.* 2007;21:836-842. Review.

Debenedectis CM, Levine D. Incidental genitourinary findings on obstetrics/gynecology ultrasound. *Ultrasound Q.* 2012;28:293-298.

Hall-Craggs MA, Kirkham A, Creighton SM. Renal and urological abnormalities occurring with Müllerian anomalies. *J Pediatr Urol.* 2011;28:27-32.

Meizner I, Yitzhak M, Levi A, Barki Y, Barnhard Y, Glezerman M. Fetal pelvic kidney: a challenge in prenatal diagnosis? *Ultrasound Obstet Gynecol.* 1995;5:391-393.

Yildirim I, Irkilata HC, Aydur E, Zor M, Basal S, Goktas S. Different clinical presentations of pelvic ectopic kidneys: report of two cases and review of the literature. *Urologia.* 2010;77:212-215. Review.

P

Polycystic Ovaries

Synonyms/Description
Polycystic ovarian syndrome (PCOS)
Stein-Leventhal syndrome

Etiology
Polycystic ovarian syndrome (PCOS) is the most common endocrine disorder in women of reproductive age, occurring in 4% to 6% of the female population. PCOS is a complex of symptoms often associated with obesity, type 2 diabetes, metabolic syndrome, and infertility. Historically there had been a lack of consensus regarding the features that define PCOS. In 2003 a consensus statement was developed between the European and American reproductive societies, known as the Rotterdam criteria, which standardized the definition of PCOS. The diagnosis requires two of the following three findings: (1) oligo-ovulation or anovulation, (2) clinical or biochemical signs of hyperandrogenism, (3) polycystic ovaries on ultrasound. It is important to note that the sonographic appearance of the ovaries is not always required for this diagnosis. The Rotterdam criteria clarify the difference between polycystic ovaries (PCO), which is a diagnostic finding, and PCOS, which is a diagnosis affecting multiple organ systems.

Ultrasound Findings
The Rotterdam sonographic definition of a PCO is the presence of either 12 or more follicles measuring 2 to 9 mm in diameter or an ovary that has an increased ovarian volume defined as greater than 10 cm³ (ovarian volume is calculated using simplified formula for prolate ellipsoid = 0.5 × length × width × thickness). Only one ovary with these findings is required with the following two exceptions.

This definition does not apply to women taking oral contraceptives.

If there is evidence of a dominant follicle (greater than 10 mm) or a corpus luteum on either ovary, the scan does not meet sonographic definition of PCO. Guidelines recommend the scan be repeated at another time (during ovarian quiescence or in the next cycle).

Differential Diagnosis
There is no differential diagnosis for a polycystic ovary when using the Rotterdam sonographic definition earlier on this page. Oral contraceptives can make the ovaries appear polycystic, and normally functioning ovaries can also appear polycystic. The ultrasound definition is limited to the appearance of the ovaries. It is important to take a clinical history in addition to the ultrasound findings so as not to overdiagnose PCOS. For example, many adolescent women have irregular menses because their hypothalamic-pituitary-ovarian axis has not yet matured, and they may have many small follicles.

Clinical Aspects and Recommendations
Ultrasound findings alone are not sufficient to diagnose or exclude PCOS in the absence of clinical information. Between 16% and 25% of the normal population have multicystic ovaries on ultrasound, but only 4% to 6% of women have polycystic ovarian syndrome. Conversely, when ultrasound reveals normal-appearing ovaries in a patient with oligo-ovulation or anovulation and hyperandrogenism, PCOS should be included in the differential diagnosis.

Patients with PCOS who are overweight should be encouraged to lose weight through diet and exercise. Drug therapies such as oral contraceptives or metformin can help with the symptoms of PCOS. PCOS may increase the risk for endometrial cancer, especially in patients with prolonged amenorrhea, because of equally long episodes of unopposed estrogen.

P

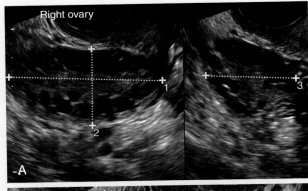

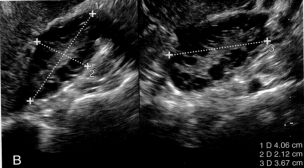

1 D 4.06 cm
2 D 2.12 cm
3 D 3.67 cm

Figure P4-1 Measurements of the right (**A**) and left (**B**) ovaries in a patient with PCOS with classic ultrasound findings.

Suggested Reading

Balen AH, Laven JSE, Tan SL, Dewailly D. Ultrasound assessment of the polycystic ovary: international consensus definitions. *Hum Reprod Update*. 2003; 9:505-514.

Polson DW, Wadsworth J, Adams J. Polycystic ovaries: a common finding in normal women. *Lancet*. 1988;1:870-872.

Wilson JF. In the clinic. The polycystic ovary syndrome. *Ann Intern Med*. 2011; 154(3): ITC2-2-ITC2-15.

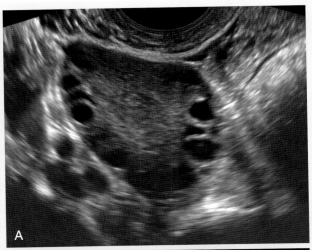

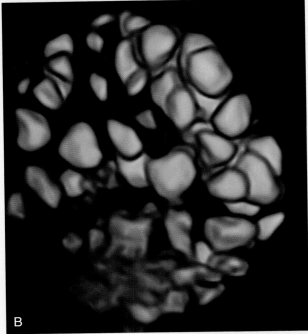

Figure P4-2 Typical polycystic ovary shown using 2-D ultrasound (**A**) and 3-D inverse mode (**B**), which shows all the individual follicles in the ovary.

Polyps, Endometrial

Synonyms/Description
None

Etiology
Endometrial polyps are relatively common intrauterine lesions that are typically benign and often asymptomatic. Hyperplastic/proliferative polyp is the most common type of polyp; it represents overgrowth of endometrial glands and stroma. Clinically they can be associated with postmenopausal and abnormal uterine bleeding as well as infertility.

Ultrasound Findings
The ultrasound appearance of endometrial polyps varies depending on whether the patient is premenopausal or postmenopausal. In premenopausal women, the endometrium (especially in the secretory/luteal phase) can be thick and heterogeneous, which often camouflages the polyps. In the proliferative/follicular phase or in postmenopausal women, when the endometrium is at its thinnest, the polyps may be more obvious because of their rounded contour and different echotexture from the surrounding endometrium. Polyps appear as hyperechoic or cystic lesions within the uterine cavity. In most cases, there is evidence of blood flow in the polyp, as seen by color flow Doppler. The stalk of the polyp can often be identified by Doppler, revealing a single-vessel pattern and thus highlighting the connection between the polyp and the underlying endometrium.

A sonohysterogram is very helpful when evaluating the endometrial cavity because polyps may not be discernible from the rest of the endometrium unless outlined by fluid.

Differential Diagnosis
When the endometrium is thickened and heterogeneous and the patient is either postmenopausal or in the proliferative/follicular phase of her cycle, a sonohysterogram may be necessary to further define the finding. If there is a small mass within the cavity, the differential diagnosis is either a polyp or a submucosal fibroid. A polyp is usually more hyperechoic than the surrounding endometrium, or it may be partly cystic. A fibroid is likely to have the same echotexture as the myometrium. Rarely, an adenomyoma can present as an intracavitary mass (see Adenomyosis). It may be difficult to differentiate a nonglobal endometrial cancer, which appears polypoid, from a true polyp.

Clinical Aspects and Recommendations
Postmenopausal patients with nonbleeding polyps are not automatic candidates for polypectomy. If it is removed, it should be done hysteroscopically, because blind D&C often misses such focal lesions. Patients with abnormal or postmenopausal bleeding are always candidates for removal of their polyps.

Increasingly, it appears that patients with asymptomatic polyps discovered incidentally need not have them automatically removed. Fernandez-Parra and colleagues reported that none of the 117 polyps removed in asymptomatic postmenopausal women were malignant. Ferrazzi and colleagues report that there was one endometrial cancer (less than 0.1%) in a polyp among 1152 asymptomatic postmenopausal women in a multicenter trial. Furthermore, Gerber and colleagues report that the detection of endometrial cancer in asymptomatic postmenopausal patients does not confer a better outcome compared with cancer patients presenting with abnormal uterine bleeding. Finally, operative hysteroscopy in such postmenopausal patients is associated with a small but significant incidence of complications (e.g., perforation, false channel, anesthesia problems).

P

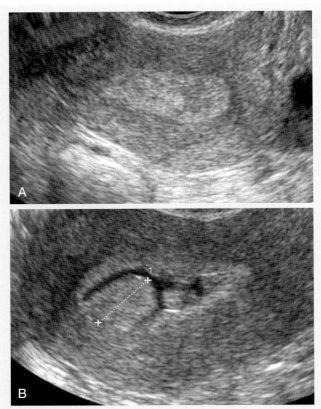

Figure P5-1   A, Patient with thickened endometrium. **B** shows that when saline is introduced into the endometrial cavity, the polyps become visible (calipers on largest one).

P

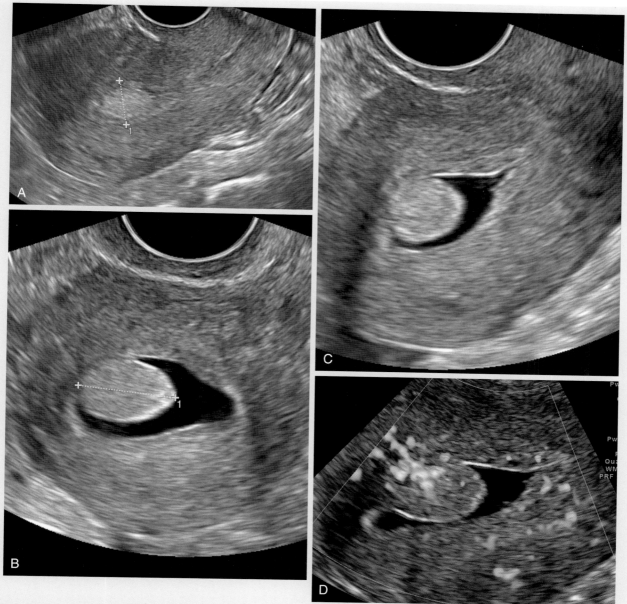

Figure P5-2 A, Thickened heterogeneous endometrium with focal echogenic area within the cavity. **B and C** show the smooth-walled polyp outlined by fluid during the sonohysterogram. **D** shows the blood flow to the polyp using color Doppler.

P

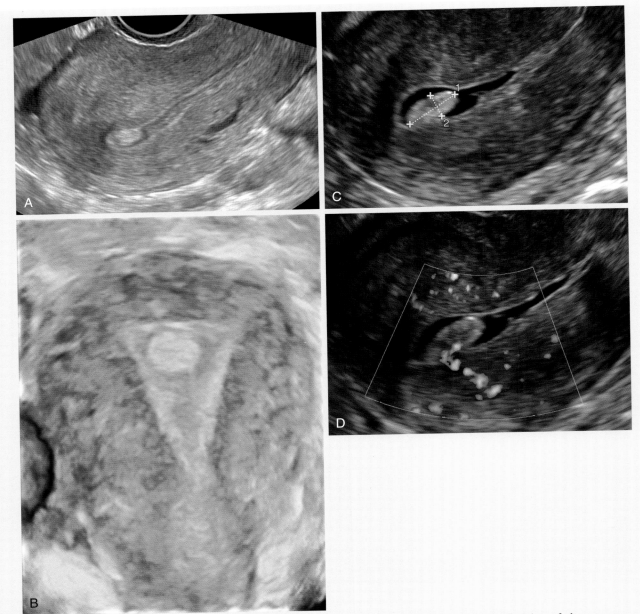

Figure P5-3 Two different patients with small 10-mm polyps seen in 2-D and 3-D at the fundus of the uterus. Note the characteristic smooth, round appearance of the polyps. **A and B** show the polyps with 2-D and 3-D transvaginal sonography. **C and D** show the polyp of a different patient using sonohysterography and color Doppler.

P

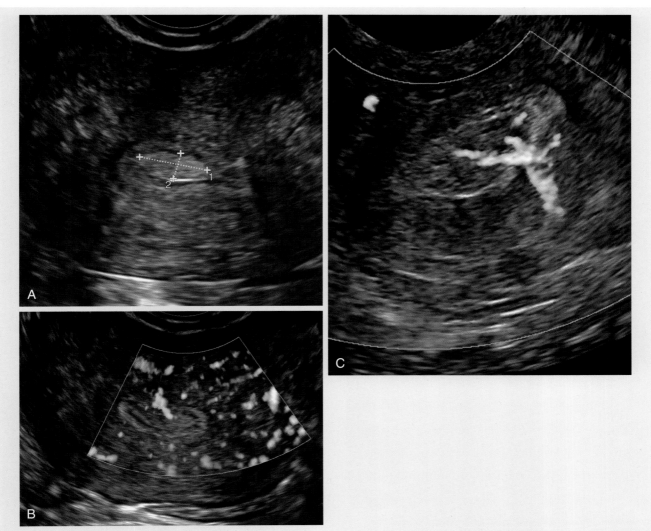

Figure P5-4 **A and B,** Small polyp *(calipers)* identified on 2-D transvaginal sonography. The diagnosis is confirmed by the presence of blood flow with a single-vessel pattern. **C** shows blood flow to a polyp in a different patient, demonstrating the similar vascular pattern.

P

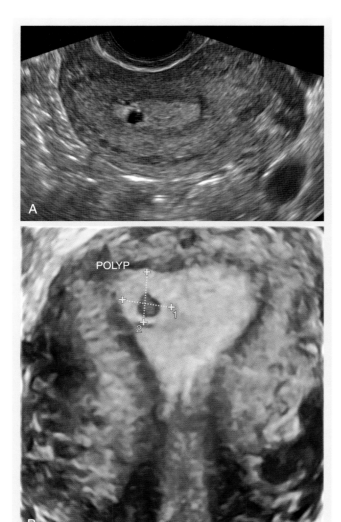

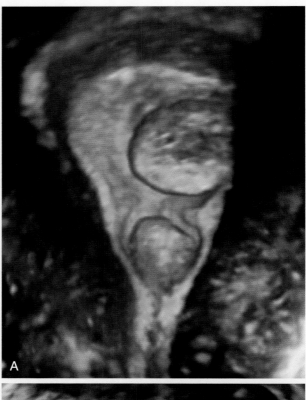

Figure P5-5   A and B, Tiny cystic polyp seen using 2-D and 3-D ultrasound, mimicking an early pregnancy. The patient was postmenopausal.

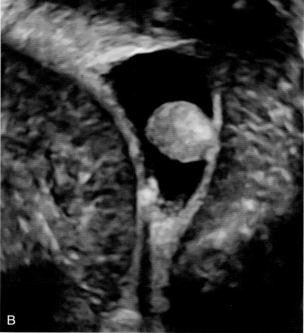

Figure P5-6   Sonohysterography with 3-D ultrasound is an excellent way to demonstrate polyps. **A and B** show two different patients with polyps.

P

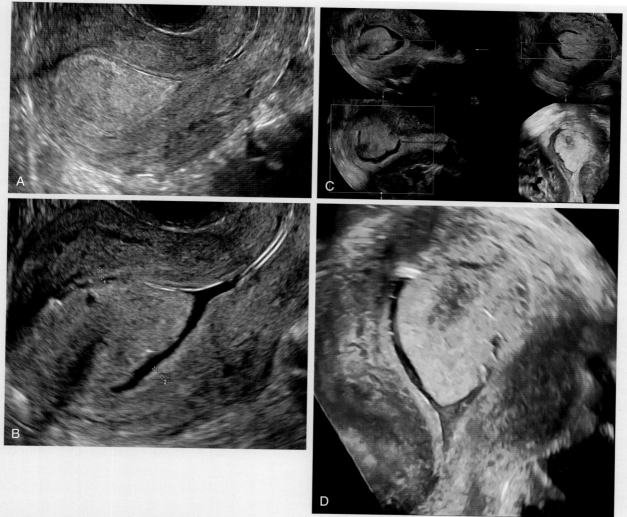

Figure P5-7   A to D, Very large polyp shown in standard 2-D **(A),** sonohysterography **(B),** and 3-D sonography with saline in the uterine cavity outlining the polyp **(C and D).**

Suggested Reading

Fang L, Su Y, Guo Y, Yingpu Sun Y. Value of 3-dimensional and power Doppler sonography for diagnosis of endometrial polyps. *Ultrasound Med.* 2013;32: 247-255.

Fernandez-Parra J, Rodriguez Oliver A, Lopez Criado S, Parrilla Fernandez F, Montoya Ventoso F. Hysteroscopic evaluation of endometrial polyps. *Int J Gynaecol Obstet.* 2006;95:144-148.

Ferrazzi E, Zupi E, Leone FP, Savelli L, Omodei U, Moscarini M, Barbieri M, Cammareri G, Capobianco G, Cicinelli E, Coccia ME, Donarini G, Fiore S, Litta P, Sideri M, Solima E, Spazzini D, Testa AC, Vignali M. How often are endometrial polyps malignant in asymptomatic postmenopausal women? A multicenter study. *Am J Obstet Gynecol.* 2009;200:235.

Gerber B, Krause A, Müller H, Reimer T, Külz T, Kundt G, Friese K. Ultrasonographic detection of asymptomatic endometrial cancer in postmenopausal patients offers no prognostic advantage over symptomatic disease discovered by uterine bleeding. *Eur J Cancer.* 2001;37:64-71.

Goldstein SR. Sonography in postmenopausal bleeding. *J Ultrasound Med.* 2012;31:333-336.

Lieng M, Istre O, Qvigstad E. Treatment of endometrial polyps: a systematic review. *Acta Obstet Gynecol.* 2010;89:992-1002.

P

Premature Ovarian Failure

Synonyms/Description
Early menopause
Ovarian insufficiency

Etiology
Premature ovarian failure (POF) occurs in women under the age of 40 and is characterized by amenorrhea, hypoestrogenism, and elevated gonadotropins. It affects an estimated 1% of women, including 0.1% under age 30. Most cases of POF are idiopathic. There are theories that POF is the result of follicular depletion, accelerated follicular atresia, or other follicular dysfunction. There are rare genetic and chromosomal causes, which generally involve the X chromosome. Other causes of POF include autoimmune oophoritis, chemotherapy or radiation, and surgical removal of the ovaries. Even a simple hysterectomy can lead to premature ovarian failure secondary to vascular disruptions.

Ultrasound Findings
The ultrasound findings in POF are indistinguishable from menopause. The ovaries tend to be small and comma-shaped, sometimes hard to locate. The uterus may also be small and will typically have a thin endometrial echo. These findings are nonspecific, and there is a large overlap between the normal appearance of the pelvis in postmenopausal patients and premenopausal patients, especially early in the follicular phase. In a study by Sokalska and Valentin, spanning 2 years before to 2 years after menopause, uterine size and left and right ovarian volumes decreased by 22%, 45%, and 20%, respectively. Two years before menopause, the total number of follicle-like cysts varied from 0 to 5, and 2 years after menopause they varied from 0 to 2.

Differential Diagnosis
The ultrasound should not be interpreted without knowing the clinical setting. There is no real differential diagnosis when seeing a normal but small uterus and ovaries, and there is no specific sonographic diagnosis for POF.

Clinical Aspects and Recommendations
The clinical symptoms of POF are similar to those of menopause, but because onset is earlier, the result is an increased risk of menopause-associated conditions such as osteoporosis and cardiovascular disease, among others. It is important that data derived on hormone therapy for menopausal patients (average age 51.4) not be blindly applied to women with POF. This is a unique population with an abnormal cessation of ovarian function, and hormone therapy in this condition has not been well studied. Adding replacement therapy until approximately age 50 will simply bring these patients back to appropriate hormone levels compared with their cohorts.

P

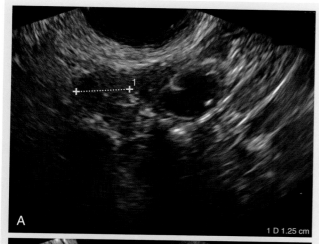

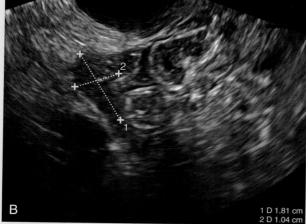

Figure P6-1 A and B, Typical comma-shaped small ovary *(calipers)* seen in patients with premature ovarian failure as well as menopause.

Suggested Reading

Kokcu A. Premature ovarian failure from current perspective. *Gynecol Endocrinol.* 2010;26:555-562.

Maclaran K, Horner E, Panay N. Premature ovarian failure: long-term sequelae. *Menopause Int.* 2010;16:38-41.

Michalakis K, Coppack SW. Primary ovarian insufficiency: relation to changes in body composition and adiposity. *Maturitas.* 2012;71:320-325.

Sokalska A, Valentin L. Changes in ultrasound morphology of the uterus and ovaries during the menopausal transition and early postmenopause: a 4-year longitudinal study. *Ultrasound Obstet Gynecol.* 2008;31:210-217.

P

R Retained Products of Conception

Synonyms/Description
RPOC
Retained placenta
Incomplete abortion

Etiology
Retained products of conception (RPOC) may occur following an abortion, a vaginal delivery, or even after a Cesarean section. This obstetric complication most commonly results in prolonged or excess vaginal bleeding and has also been associated with endometritis. The retained tissue may include a portion of the placenta (such as a succenturiate lobe) or tissue from a pregnancy not completely evacuated.

Ultrasound Findings
Retained products of conception typically appear as an echogenic, vascular mass with ill-defined borders, centrally located within the endometrial cavity. The mass may contain areas of fluid but is largely solid. Color Doppler often shows an alarming amount of vascularity, which has been described as mimicking an arteriovenous malformation (AVM); however, this resolves completely after evacuation of the retained products. The sonographic appearance of the retained tissue can have characteristics of placenta, especially if the patient is postpartum. If the patient had an early pregnancy loss or termination, the tissue is more often echogenic with small cystic areas. Abundant vascularity is a characteristic feature of most types of retained products of conception.

Durfee and colleagues report that an endometrial mass is the most sensitive (79%) and specific (89%) sonographic finding in patients with retained products of conception. None of the patients in their study with this diagnosis had a completely normal scan.

Regarding vascularity, Atri and colleagues report that the presence of focal vascularity had sensitivity, specificity, negative predictive value, and positive predictive value of 94%, 67%, 95%, and 65%, respectively. Of the patients with pathologically confirmed retained products of conception, five had focal increased vascularity without a mass, but none had a mass without focal increased vascularity.

Differential Diagnosis
When observing a vascular mass in the endometrium, it is important to determine the clinical history. The sonographic appearance alone may suggest a large polyp or an abnormal endometrium such as hyperplasia or endometrial cancer. If the vascularity in the lesion is dramatic, an AVM may be suspected, although primary uterine AVMs are exceedingly rare. If the patient is postpartum or if there has been a recent pregnancy loss, the diagnosis is retained products of conception until proved otherwise.

Clinical Aspects and Recommendations
In patients who have had a first trimester pregnancy loss or termination, the presence of vascularity may be helpful in predicting the success of expectant management for RPOC. In the study by Casikar and colleagues, the absence of color flow was predictive of successful expectant management with a sensitivity, specificity, positive predictive value, negative predictive value, and positive likelihood ratio of 90.3%, 37.5%, 89%, 40.9%, and 1.445, respectively. There was no correlation between the volume of the retained products and the success of expectant management.

Active management includes both surgical and medical options. Medical management with misoprostol, a prostaglandin agonist, is a relatively new tool. Treatment with misoprostol for retained products from early pregnancy failure showed a greater than 90% success rate in women presenting with localized abdominal pain, Rh-negative blood type, or a combination of active bleeding and nulliparity. Thus, in a select group, the decision to pursue expectant, medical, or surgical management depends on multiple factors, including patient preference. Patients presenting with hemodynamically symptomatic bleeding or acute hemorrhage require surgical management with dilation and curettage (D&C). In these patients, swift action is needed to remove the cause of bleeding since such patients can rapidly develop disseminated intravascular coagulopathy (DIC).

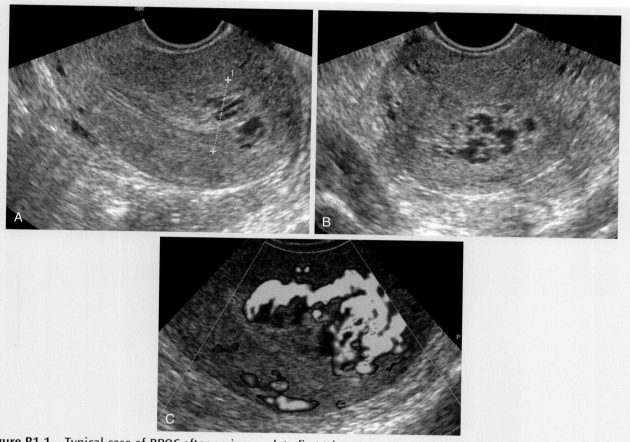

Figure R1-1 Typical case of RPOC after an incomplete first trimester pregnancy loss. **A and B** (gray-scale views) show the ill-defined margins of the endometrium at the fundus with irregular cystic spaces. The color Doppler in **C** shows that these spaces are blood vessels in this very vascular case of RPOC.

R

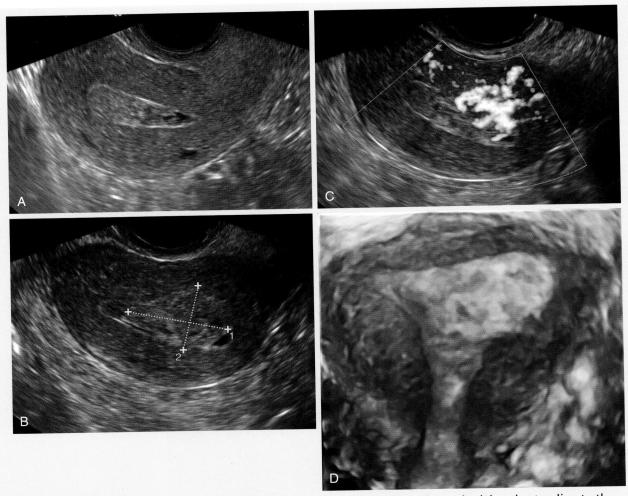

Figure R1-2   A to D, The uterine cavity contains an echogenic mass, filling the cavity (**A**) and extending to the edge of the endometrium, blurring the margins (**B,** *calipers*). **C** shows the abundant color flow at the site of the RPOC. **D** shows the 3-D appearance of the same case, demonstrating an asymmetric enlargement and deformity of the left fundus/cornu, representing the RPOC.

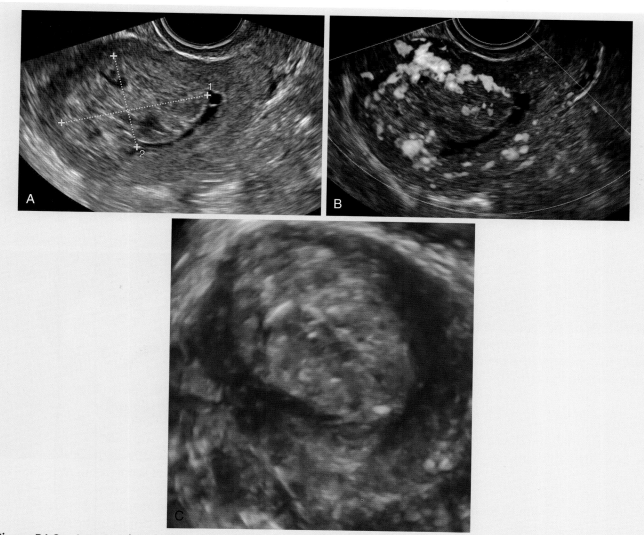

Figure R1-3   A to C, Sclerotic RPOC, 6 months after a term delivery (2-D, Doppler, and 3-D images). Note the complex-appearing vascular mass involving the endometrium. If this were seen in a postmenopausal patient with bleeding, the appearance would be consistent with endometrial cancer. The history of a symptomatic postpartum patient enabled the correct diagnosis of longstanding RPOC (sclerotic on pathologic examination).

R

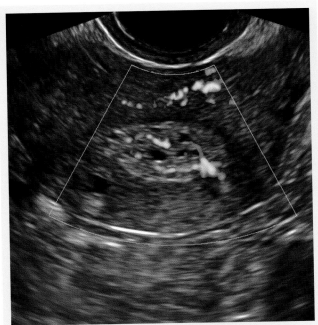

Figure R1-4   Patient with an endometrial polyp. Note the similarity to the RPOCs. This patient had never been pregnant

Videos
Videos 1 and 2 on retained products of contraception are available online.

Suggested Reading
Atri M, Rao A, Boylan C, Rasty G, Gerber D. Best predictors of grayscale ultrasound combined with color Doppler in the diagnosis of retained products of conception. *J Clin Ultrasound.* 2011;39:122-127.

Casikar I, Lu C, Oates J, Bignardi T, Alhamdan D, Condous G. The use of power Doppler colour scoring to predict successful expectant management in women with an incomplete miscarriage. *Hum Reprod.* 2011;27:669-675.

Creinin MD, Huang X, Gilles J, Barnhart K, Westhoff C, Zhang J. Medical management of early pregnancy failure. *Obstet Gynecol.* 2006;107:901-907.

Durfee SM, Frates MC, Luong A, Benson CB. The sonographic and color Doppler features of retained products of conception. *J Ultrasound Med.* 2005; 24:1181-1186.

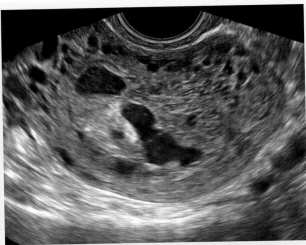

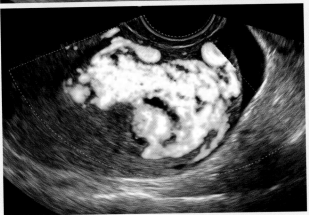

Figure R1-5   Rare case of spontaneous AVM unrelated to pregnancy. The entire uterus is replaced by cystic areas on gray-scale imaging. Color flow Doppler shows abnormal vessels reaching to the serosa and involving much of the myometrium. The pattern and clinical history were very different in this nulliparous patient.

Scarred Uterus and Asherman's Syndrome

S

Synonyms/Description

Intrauterine adhesions or synechiae

Etiology

Most cases of intrauterine adhesions result from trauma to the endometrium, primarily from dilation and curettage (D&C) procedures. Patients most at risk for developing Asherman's syndrome are those undergoing D&C postpartum for retained products of conception, incomplete spontaneous abortion (SAB), or therapeutic abortion (TAB). Intrauterine synechiae can occur after any procedure or process that causes trauma to the normal endometrium. Examples in addition to those discussed include abdominal or hysteroscopic myomectomy, hysteroscopic septoplasty, and previous placenta accreta, among others. Synechiae are connective tissue bands that disrupt the endometrium, causing a lack of distention of the uterine cavity. They are associated with recurrent pregnancy loss and infertility.

Schenker and Margalioth studied 1856 cases of Asherman's syndrome and showed that pregnancy was the main predisposing factor in 90.8% of the patients, with 66.7% of cases occurring after D&C for SAB or TAB, 21.5% after postpartum D&C, 2% after Cesarean section, and 0.6% after evacuation of trophoblastic disease.

These results appear to show that the endometrium is most vulnerable to developing Asherman's syndrome during the hypoestrogenic state immediately after pregnancy.

Asherman's syndrome may also occur after endometrial ablation. These procedures aim to destroy the basalis layer of the endometrium to decrease menstrual bleeding. If synechiae occur, it makes subsequent evaluation of any abnormal bleeding extremely difficult.

Ultrasound Findings

In patients with Asherman's syndrome, the endometrial echo is difficult to see, with irregular borders and disruptions of the endometrial lining in multiple areas. There may also be small, focal, cystic-like areas containing blood within the endometrial cavity, trapped by the adhesions. Using 3-D ultrasound, the outline of the endometrial cavity is irregular, shaggy, and distorted. Linear adhesions are usually seen, traversing the endometrium, leaving small islands of endometrial echo.

The most accurate method for diagnosing Asherman's syndrome is sonohysterography, in which saline is injected into the uterine cavity through a small catheter threaded through the cervix. In severe cases, it may not be possible to distend the cavity at all, thus confirming the diagnosis of extensive adhesions. The adhesions may be seen sonographically traversing the cavity in patients when saline can distend the cavity even slightly.

Differential Diagnosis

The clinical history is essential in making the diagnosis of Asherman's syndrome. A likely scenario is a patient presenting with infertility and amenorrhea whose history is significant for a D&C following her last pregnancy.

The ill-defined endometrial echo may suggest the diagnosis of adenomyosis, although in that case the uterus is typically globular and asymmetric, which is not usually a feature of Asherman's syndrome. Fibroids or polyps can also distort the endometrium, but these patients typically complain of excess bleeding, unlike patients with intrauterine adhesions, who are more likely to present with amenorrhea or oligomenorrhea.

It is remotely possible that a thick synechia could be confused with a uterine septum, although it is unlikely because of the asymmetry of adhesions compared with septa.

Clinical Aspects and Recommendations

Patients with significant Asherman's syndrome are usually infertile and amenorrheic. They are typically treated with hysteroscopic lysis of adhesions, sometimes with intrauterine "stenting," followed by treatment with sequential estrogen and progesterone therapy to repair the endometrium.

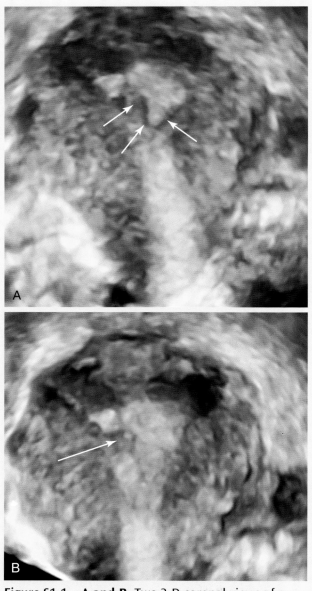

Figure S1-1   A and B, Two 3-D coronal views of a patient with Asherman's syndrome. Note the echolucent linear jagged structures (adhesions; *arrows*) traversing the endometrial cavity.

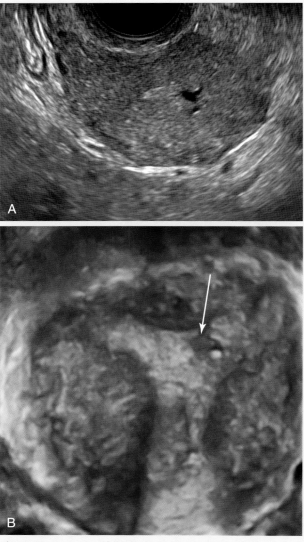

Figure S1-2   A and B, 2-D and 3-D views of a severely scarred *(arrows)* endometrium in a patient who had recurrent SABs and D&C's.

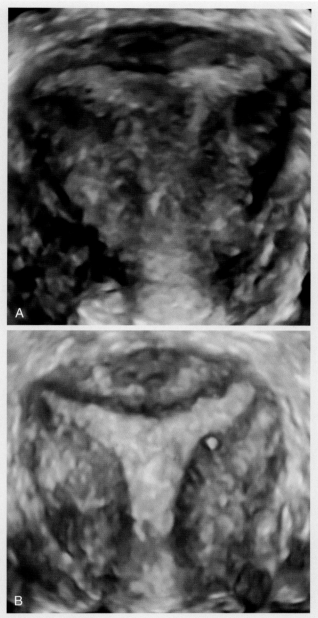

Figure S1-3   A, 3-D coronal view of the shaggy endometrial cavity in a patient with Asherman's syndrome and infertility. **B** is a similar view of the same uterus after hysteroscopic surgery for lysis of the adhesions. Note that the margins of the endometrium are sharper and smoother than preoperatively.

S

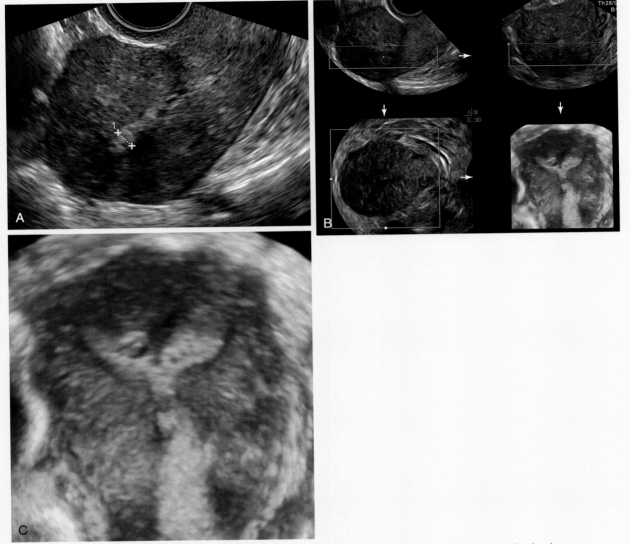

Figure S1-4   A to C, 2-D, multiplanar, and 3-D rendering of the uterine cavity in a patient who had an endometrial ablation because of excessive vaginal bleeding. Note the irregular outline and severe scarring of the margins of the cavity; this should not be confused with a partial septum.

S

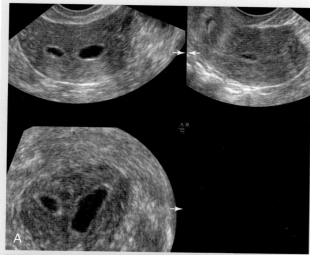

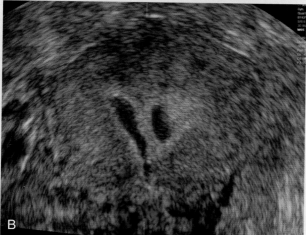

Figure S1-5 A and B, Two different patients with uterine synechiae seen during a sonohysterogram. Note the fluid outlining the adhesion within the uterine cavity. These adhesions are similar in appearance to a uterine septum, although correctly diagnosed because of asymmetry.

Suggested Reading

Berman JM. Intrauterine adhesions. *Semin Reprod Med.* 2008;26:349-355.

Knopman J, Copperman AB. Value of 3D ultrasound in the management of suspected Asherman's syndrome. *J Reprod Med.* 2007;52:1016-1022.

Schenker JG, Margalioth EJ. Intrauterine adhesions: an updated appraisal. *Fertil Steril.* 1982;37:593-610.

Yu D, Wong YM, Cheong Y, Xia E, Li TC. Asherman syndrome—one century later. *Fertil Steril.* 2008;89:759-779.

Schwannoma

S

Synonyms/Description
Schwann cell tumor

Etiology
Schwannomas are peripheral nerve sheath tumors composed of Schwann cells, which produce myelin that covers and insulates nerve fibers. Schwannomas can occur in isolation or may be associated with neurofibromatosis type I (previously known as von Recklinghausen's disease).

Nerve sheath tumors can occur anywhere along the peripheral nervous system, with only 3% of Schwannomas arising in the retroperitoneum and pelvis. Retroperitoneal Schwannomas tend to be very large when detected because they are usually asymptomatic or associated with nonspecific symptoms, thus delaying diagnosis. Malignant peripheral nerve sheath tumors are even more rare and are classified as sarcomas.

Ultrasound Findings
Schwannomas are typically solid, hypoechoic, and well encapsulated, sometimes with cystic areas and calcifications. They can grow large, up to 20 cm in diameter, and tend to be vascular, often with central hemorrhage and infarction. The appearance is nonspecific, making the correct diagnosis by imaging difficult. The large masses often displace normal retroperitoneal structures such as the kidney and ureter without invading them.

Differential Diagnosis
The differential diagnosis includes any solid or complex vascular mass that is large, posterior (retroperitoneal), and displacing other organs. This includes sarcomas, lymphomas, neurofibromas, metastatic disease, renal cell carcinoma, and other retroperitoneal tumors. When present in the pelvic area (presacral), they may be confused with degenerating fibroids, although the lack of a uterine stalk should argue against a fibroid.

Clinical Aspects and Recommendations
Schwannomas are typically benign and only treated when symptomatic. Malignant Schwannomas are classified as sarcomas and typically are very aggressive. These are managed by multidisciplinary teams, which include surgeons, oncologists, and other specialists.

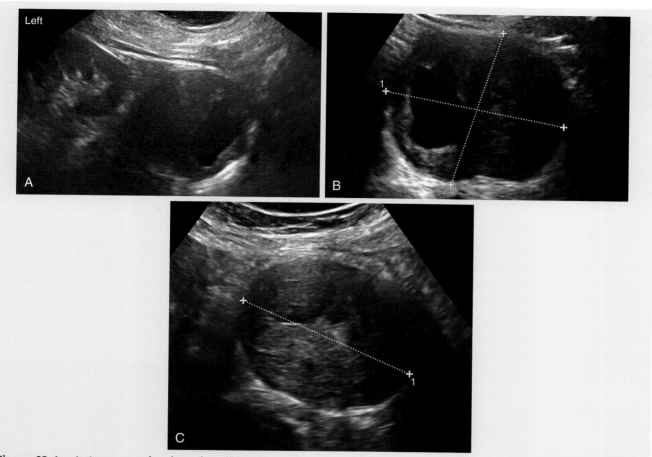

Figure S2-1 **A,** Large, predominantly solid tumor with an irregular cystic component, located high in the adnexa, just below the inferior pole of the left kidney. **B and C** show two different views of the mass, demonstrating the smooth outer border and the solid texture with cystic spaces.

Suggested Reading

Daneshmand S, Youssefzadeh D, Chamie K, Boswell W, Wu N, Stein JP, Boyd S, Skinner DG. Benign retroperitoneal schwannoma: a case series and review of the literature. *Urology.* 2003;62:993-997.

Habib T, Hamdi JT, Hussain W, Almiamini W, Hamdi K, Wani AM, Al Zeyani NR. Presacral schwannoma treated as irritable bowel syndrome. *BMJ Case Rep.* 2010; 2010:pii.

Kudo T, Kawakami H, Kuwatani M, Ehira N, Yamato H, Eto K, Kubota K, Asaka M. Three cases of retroperitoneal schwannoma diagnosed by EUS-FNA. *World J Gastroenterol.* 2011;17:3459-3464.

Serous Cystadenoma

Synonyms/Description

An epithelial-stromal cystic tumor containing serous fluid

Etiology

Serous cystadenomas are the most common type of epithelial-stromal tumors. They are lined with cells similar to those lining the fallopian tubes, suggesting that the origin may be tubal rather than ovarian. These cysts can become very large, although not typically as large as mucinous cystadenomas, and up to 20% are bilateral. Most (70%) are benign, whereas 5% to 10% have borderline malignant potential, and 20% to 25% are frankly malignant, although there is no indication that benign serous tumors transform into malignant ones.

Ultrasound Findings

Serous cystadenomas are typically thin-walled unilocular cysts, although they can also be multilocular. They are filled with serous fluid, which is usually clear or may contain tiny particles. Although less common, a borderline or malignant tumor must be considered (see elsewhere in the book for more information on borderline and malignant ovarian tumors) in cysts with solid components or nodules, especially if blood flow is detected with color Doppler.

Differential Diagnosis

The differential diagnosis includes any adnexal cystic mass such as a mucinous cystadenoma, cystadenofibroma, endometrioma, peritoneal inclusion cyst, degenerating fibroid, or hydrosalpinx. When unilocular, or simple, they are virtually indistinguishable from functional type follicular cysts. The presence of a separate ovary may be helpful to focus on non-ovarian etiologies such as a hydrosalpinx, degenerating fibroid, or even paraovarian cysts. A mucinous cystadenoma is more likely to be multicystic, displaying varying sonographic textures within the different compartments compared with a serous cystadenoma. An endometrioma typically has characteristic homogeneous low-level echoes. Serous cystadenomas and some cystadenofibromas can be virtually indistinguishable.

Clinical Aspects and Recommendations

Cysts that are symptomatic, growing over several cycles, or extremely large are typically managed surgically. The type of surgery and route will depend on multiple factors, such as the patient's age, reproductive stage, size of the mass, and benign versus nonbenign appearance of the mass.

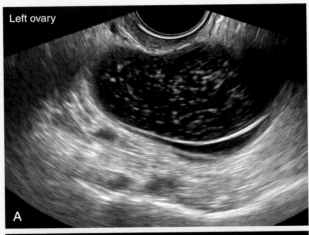

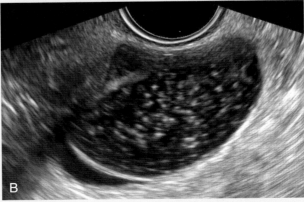

Figure S3-1 **A and B,** Unilocular serous cystadenoma of the left ovary. Note that there are no solid areas or nodularity.

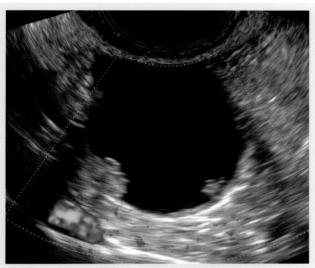

Figure S3-2 Serous cystadenoma with small areas of nodularity but no internal blood flow. This is indistinguishable sonographically from a cystadenofibroma.

Suggested Reading

Maheshwari V, Tyagi SP, Saxena K, Tyagi N, Sharma R, Aziz M, Hameed F. Surface epithelial tumours of the ovary. *Indian J Pathol Microbiol.* 1994;37:75-85.

Sujatha VV, Babu SC. Giant ovarian serous cystadenoma in a postmenopausal woman: a case report. *Cases J.* 2009;2:7875.

S

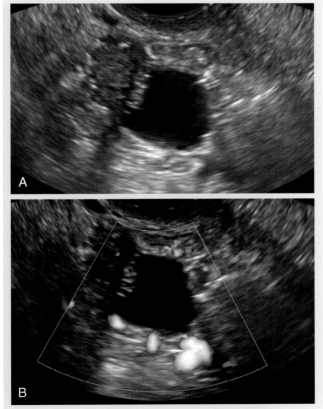

Figure S3-3 A and B, Small paraovarian serous cystadenoma. Similar to Figure S2-2, this lesion has some mural irregularities but without detectable blood flow.

Struma Ovarii

Synonyms/Description
Monodermal, highly specialized mature cystic teratoma comprised of ectopic thyroid tissue

Etiology
Struma ovarii is an extremely rare condition. It is defined as the presence of thyroid tissue comprising greater than 50% of the cellular component in an ovarian tumor, virtually always a teratoma. Struma ovarii is a mature teratoma and accounts for approximately 3% of all ovarian teratomas. It is usually benign, although 5% have malignant components that can occasionally metastasize. Tumors may have features of a multinodular goiter, with colloid nodules and hyperplastic changes. These tumors can vary in size, but most are greater than 5 cm at diagnosis.

Ultrasound Findings
The typical sonographic appearance of struma ovarii is similar to that of a dermoid cyst with one or more echogenic nodules known as struma pearls. Although the echogenic nodules in dermoids have no evidence of color flow on Doppler interrogation, the struma pearl may be quite vascular, which is a valuable clue to the correct diagnosis. Sonographically, most cases of struma ovarii are nonspecific in appearance and are largely solid or have both cystic and solid portions. Less commonly, the tumor is predominantly or entirely cystic, although most of these are multilocular. Occasionally, struma ovarii will have a unilocular cystic appearance, making a specific sonographic diagnosis difficult.

Doppler is very helpful in detecting struma ovarii because most are vascular and demonstrate more blood flow than typically seen in a dermoid cyst.

Up to 17% of patients with benign struma ovarii may have ascites. Struma ovarii may be associated with a contralateral dermoid or other types of teratoma.

There are no specific sonographic features that help distinguish malignant from benign struma ovarii tumors.

Differential Diagnosis
Struma ovarii can mimic a dermoid cyst, although presence of Doppler flow in the solid portions is very helpful to distinguish a struma ovarii from a dermoid. Because struma ovarii can be solid, solid and cystic, or completely cystic with or without septations, the appearance is nonspecific and makes a precise diagnosis almost impossible. Struma ovarii can also masquerade as an endometrioma, other types of teratomas, or essentially any ovarian malignancy, depending on the degree of flow demonstrated by Doppler.

Clinical Aspects and Recommendations
They are most commonly seen in reproductive-age women; however, incidence peaks between the ages of 40 and 60. The possible presence of struma ovarii should be suspected in a woman with hyperthyroidism who has no goiter and minimal thyroid uptake of radioactive iodine. Even among such women, however, true struma ovarii is rare.

Treatment of hyperthyroidism associated with struma ovarii consists primarily of surgical excision, mainly because of the risk of carcinoma. In those patients who are symptomatic or have substantial serologic evidence of hyperthyroidism, use of an antithyroid drug for 4 to 6 weeks before surgery is recommended. The cyst should be removed surgically.

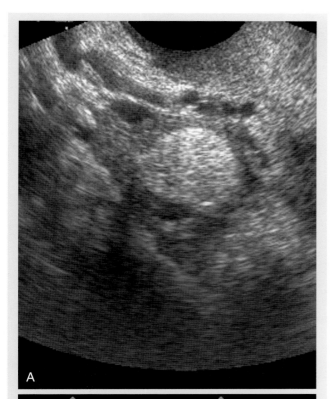

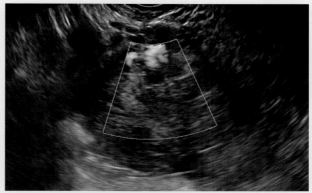

Figure S4-2 Struma ovarii presenting as a large, solid, heterogenous mass with several areas of relative increase in echogenicity. Note the presence of blood flow in the mass.

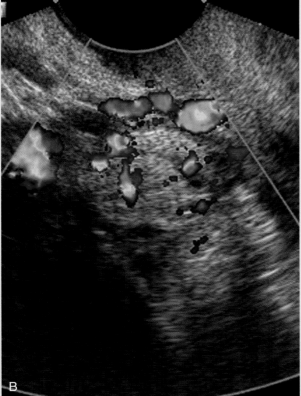

Figure S4-1 **A,** Small echogenic mass whose appearance suggests a dermoid. **B,** Doppler color flow with moderate vascularity in the mass, a characteristic of struma ovarii.

S

S

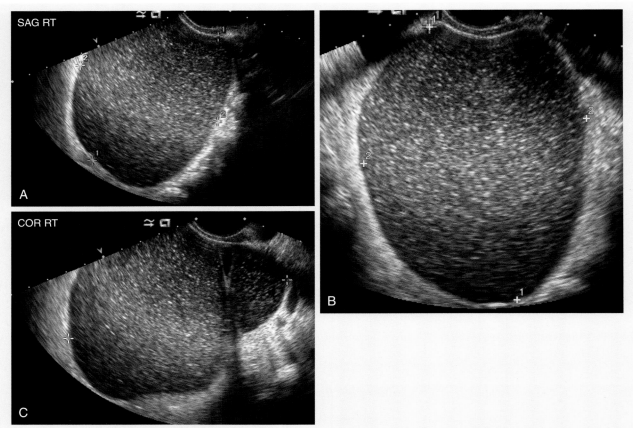

Figure S4-3   A to C, Struma ovarii presenting as a large 8-cm cystic mass with a few septations. The cystic portions have dense, homogeneous echoes and no blood flow. Although the pattern of internal echoes might suggest an endometrioma, the internal echoes are too coarse.

Suggested Reading

Coyne C, Nikiforov YE. RAS mutation-positive follicular variant of papillary thyroid carcinoma arising in a struma ovarii. *Endocr Pathol.* 2010;21:144-147.

Doganay M, Gungor T, Cavkaytar S, Sirvan L, Mollamahmutoglu L. Malignant struma ovarii with a focus of papillary thyroid cancer: a case report. *Arch Gynecol Obstet.* 2008;277:371-373.

Manini C, Magistris A, Puopolo M, Montironi PL. Cystic struma ovarii: a report of three cases. *Pathologica.* 2010;102:36-38.

Saba L, Guerriero S, Sulcis R, Virgilio B, Melis G, Mallarini G. Mature and immature ovarian teratomas: CT, US and MR imaging characteristics. *Eur J Radiol.* 2009;72:454-463.

Zalel Y, Seidman DS, Oren M, Achiron R, Gotlieb W, Mashiach S, Goldenberg M. Sonographic and clinical characteristics of struma ovarii. *J Ultrasound Med.* 2000;19:857-861.

T-Shaped Uterus

Synonyms/Description
T-shaped uterus refers to the imaging appearance of a T rather than a triangular-shaped endometrial cavity

Etiology
Diethylstilbestrol (DES) is a synthetic estrogen that was widely prescribed to pregnant women from the late 1940s until 1970 to prevent miscarriage. An estimated 1 million to 1.5 million women received DES during their pregnancies, and this ultimately affected the reproductive organs of 35% to 69% of their female offspring. The daughters of women treated with DES developed congenital malformations of the uterus, cervix, and vagina as well as adenosis and (rarely) clear cell adenocarcinoma of the vagina. The T-shaped uterus is the most common and characteristic deformity of the uterus resulting from the prenatal exposure to DES and is highly associated with infertility and recurrent miscarriage.

Initially, the term "T-shaped uterus" was reserved for the DES daughters with the characteristic uterine cavity shape. More recently, patients with multiple D&Cs or hysteroscopic procedures can develop endometrial scarring that can be very similar in appearance and outcome to the congenital T-shaped uterus. Sometimes a patient may have recurrent miscarriages and D&Cs with a subsequent diagnosis of T-shaped uterus as a result of Asherman's syndrome. Whether those patients had a congenital T-shaped uterus or acquired extensive scarring that distorted the endometrial cavity often cannot be determined.

Ultrasound Findings
The exact shape of the uterine cavity is usually not discernible on a standard 2-D ultrasound. The coronal view of the uterus, usually reconstructed from a 3-D volume, is necessary to evaluate the shape of the uterus and endometrial cavity.

A normal uterine cavity is triangular or V-shaped, with the three apices being the two cornua and the junction of the lower uterine segment and the cervix (level of internal os). When the uterus is T-shaped, there is a waist in the sides of the triangle such that the corpus of the endometrial cavity is narrowed and takes on the shape of a T rather than a V. The outer myometrial surface of the uterus (the serosal surface) is typically unaffected.

Differential Diagnosis
The differential diagnosis of a T-shaped uterine cavity relates more to the cause, such as Asherman's syndrome and uterine scarring versus congenital anomaly (see Scarred Uterus and Asherman's Syndrome and also Müllerian Duct Anomalies).Occasionally a fibroid can press on the uterine cavity, creating the appearance of a T shape because of the location of the fibroid. Other congenital Müllerian duct abnormalities are usually characteristic, such as a septate or unicornuate uterus, and quite different from a T-shaped cavity.

Clinical Aspects and Recommendations
Women found to have a T-shaped endometrial cavity are best managed by specialists in infertility, hysteroscopic surgery, and high-risk obstetrics.

Fernandez and colleagues studied 97 infertile women who had T-shaped uteri, and 49.5% of them became pregnant after metroplasty. For these patients, the pregnancy rate increased from 0% to 73%, and their miscarriage rate fell from 78% to 27% ($p = 0.05$). For all 57 pregnancies in 48 women, the preterm delivery rate was 14%, the term delivery rate was 49%, and the live birth rate was 63%.

In another study by Katz and colleagues, which included eight patients with T-shaped uteri and recurrent miscarriage, hysteroscopic surgery resulted in four term pregnancies in three women, one ectopic pregnancy, and no abortions.

T

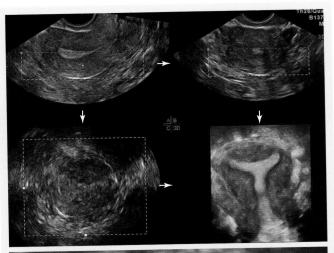

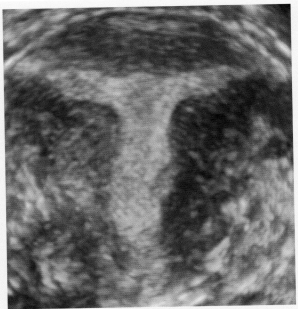

Figure T1-2   Classic T-shaped uterus in a DES daughter who was never able to conceive.

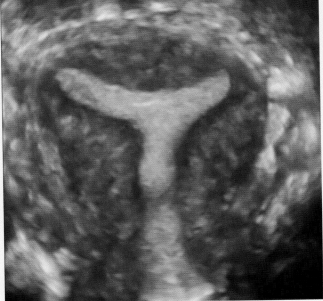

Figure T1-1   3-D image of a T-shaped uterus in a patient with recurrent miscarriage. Note the lack of triangular shape of the lateral walls of the endometrial cavity. Instead, the lateral walls are pulled inward to create a T configuration, thus narrowing the cavity. The outer uterine surface, however, is normally shaped, as is expected with this diagnosis.

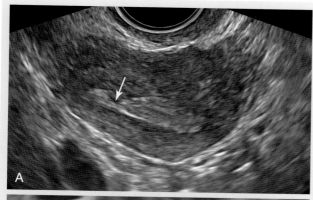

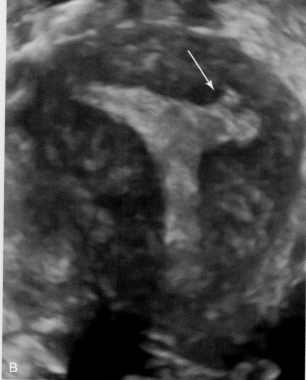

Figure T1-3   A and B, 2-D and 3-D images of the uterus in a patient with multiple D&Cs. Note that although the shape is slightly T-shaped, the main abnormality is scarring *(arrows)* and irregularity of the left cornu with asymmetry of the shape of the uterine cavity.

Suggested Reading

Fernandez H, Garbin O, Castaigne V, Gervaise A, Levaillant JM. Surgical approach to and reproductive outcome after surgical correction of a T-shaped uterus. *Hum Reprod.* 2011;26(7):1730-1734.

Katz Z, Ben-Arie A, Lurie S, Manor M, Insler V. Beneficial effect of hysteroscopic metroplasty on the reproductive outcome in a 'T-shaped' uterus. *Gynecol Obstet Invest.* 1996;41(1):41-43.

van Gils AP, Tham RT, Falke TH, Peters AA. Abnormalities of the uterus and cervix after diethylstilbestrol exposure: correlation of findings on MR and hysterosalpingography. *AJR Am J Roentgenol.* 1989;153(6):1235-1238.

T

Tarlov Cysts

Synonyms/Description
Perineural cysts

Etiology
These perineural cysts are of unknown etiology and arise in sacral nerve roots, in an extradural location and communicate with the thecal sac. They are seen on pelvic ultrasound when they extend through adjacent foramina with erosion of the bone. These cysts are often multiple and bilateral. They are usually an incidental finding on asymptomatic patients, although they may cause pelvic or lower back pain.

Ultrasound Findings
The sonographic appearance of Tarlov cysts includes cystic masses (often bilateral) in the posterior part of the pelvis, fixed to the pelvic side wall. Careful scanning will reveal that the uterus and ovaries are separate from these masses, which lie along the posterior pelvic side wall. Tarlov cysts are avascular on color Doppler.

Differential Diagnosis
It is important to visualize the ovaries separately from these cysts; otherwise, it is easy to mistake them for endometriomas, hydrosalpinges, ectopic pregnancy, lymphadenopathy (lymphoma), or retroperitoneal sarcoma. These entities all have the sonographic appearance of complex cystic masses, often bilateral and sometimes solid-looking because of their internal echoes. Because Tarlov cysts are found in the posterior compartment of the pelvis, the practitioner needs to consider this diagnosis and seek out separate ovaries to arrive at the correct diagnosis.

Clinical Aspects and Recommendations
Treatment is undertaken for symptomatic patients with perineural cysts and may involve surgery with sacral laminectomy and cyst removal. Microsurgical cyst fenestration and CT-guided percutaneous cyst aspiration have also been undertaken, but the fluid tends to reaccumulate after aspiration.

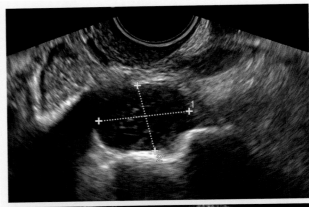
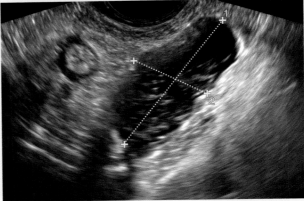

Figure T2-1 Bilateral posterior adnexal masses—proven Tarlov cysts in two different patients.

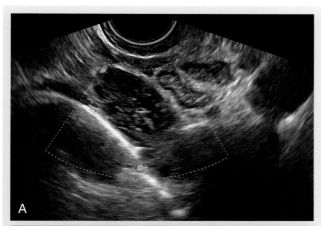

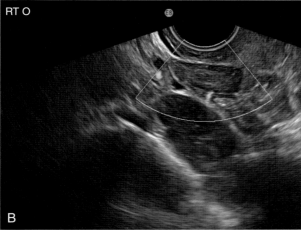

Figure T2-2 The same patient as in the top image of Figure T2-1. **A,** Note the lack of blood flow in the mass. **B** shows the normal ovary anterior to the mass.

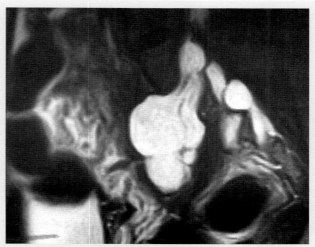

Figure T2-3 MRI in a different patient—typical appearance of Tarlov cyst extending anteriorly from neural foramina. *(With permission* J Ultrasound Med. *1994;13:803-805.)*

Suggested Reading

H'ng MW, Wanigasiri UI, Ong CL. Perineural (Tarlov) cysts mimicking adnexal masses: a report of three cases. *Ultrasound Obstet Gynecol.* 2009;34:230-233.

McClure MJ, Atri M, Haider MA, Murphy J. Perineural cysts presenting as complex adnexal cystic masses on transvaginal sonography. *AJR Am J Roentgenol.* 2001;177:1313-1318.

Mummaneni PV, Pitts LH, McCormack BM, Corroo JM, Weinstein PR. Microsurgical treatment of symptomatic sacral Tarlov cysts. *Neurosurgery.* 2000; 47:74-78.

Raza S, Klapholz H, Benacerraf BR. Tarlov cysts: a cause of bilateral adnexal masses on pelvic sonography. *J Ultrasound Med.* 1994;13:803-805.

Theca Lutein Cyst

Synonyms/Description
Hyperreactio luteinalis

Etiology
Theca lutein cysts are benign, functional cysts of pregnancy. They are usually multiple, bilateral, and large. The exact etiology is unknown but is associated with high circulating levels of (or an increased sensitivity to) human chorionic gonadotropin (hCG), the "hormone of pregnancy." They are typically seen in patients with trophoblastic disease, with multiple pregnancy, or who have undergone infertility treatment (ovarian stimulation followed by pregnancy). Up to 50% of patients with molar pregnancies and 10% of patients with choriocarcinoma develop theca lutein cysts. Occasionally, theca lutein cysts can occur in pregnancies associated with large placentas, such as those affected with diabetes or Rh sensitization. Rarely, they can also occur in normal, singleton pregnancies.

Ultrasound Findings
Theca lutein cysts are large, usually bilateral, adnexal masses that consist of many thin-walled smaller cystic components, giving them the appearance of a "spoke wheel." The cystic components are typically anechoic, although focal hemorrhage can occur, demonstrated as internal echoes. Bilateral, multiple, predominantly clear, large cysts in a pregnant patient should be highly suggestive of theca lutein cysts. Color Doppler should be considered to exclude torsion since these patients are at increased risk.

Differential Diagnosis
Although there is a vast differential diagnosis, including many benign ovarian tumors, the presence of bilateral symmetric, anechoic cysts with the characteristic spoke-wheel appearance in a pregnant patient is virtually pathognomonic for theca lutein cysts.

Clinical Aspects and Recommendations
Theca lutein cysts are functional cysts, which are usually asymptomatic and spontaneously resolve during pregnancy or in the postpartum period. Intervention is only indicated if they become symptomatic and conservative management is not an option. These masses increase the risk of ovarian torsion; if suspected, they require immediate surgical management. Theca lutein cysts can occur in patients with gestational trophoblastic disease, in which the treatment should be based on the trophoblastic tumor rather than the accompanying cysts.

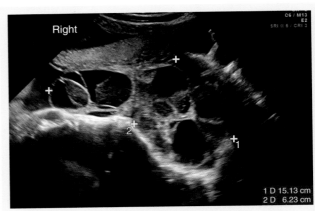

Figure T3-1 Markedly enlarged right ovary in a pregnant patient previously treated with ovulation-induction drugs. The contralateral ovary was similar in appearance. Note that a few of the cystic spaces contain clots consistent with focal areas of hemorrhage.

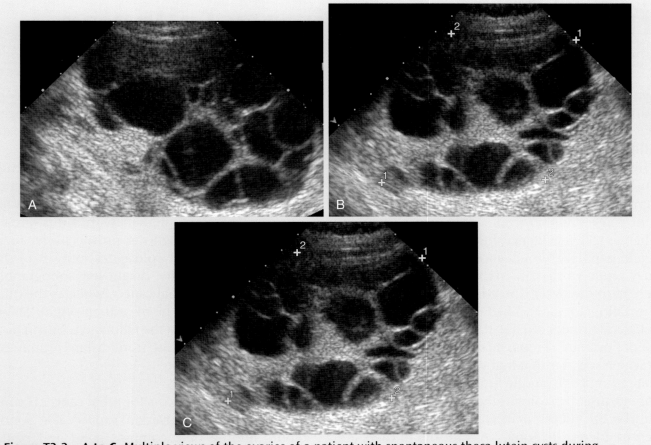

Figure T3-2   A to C, Multiple views of the ovaries of a patient with spontaneous theca lutein cysts during pregnancy.

Suggested Reading

Amoah C, Yassin A, Cockayne E, Bird A. Hyperreactio luteinalis in pregnancy. *Fertil Steril.* 2011;95:24-29.

Holsbeke C, Amant F, Veldman J, de Boodt A, Merman P, Timmerman D. Hyperreactio luteinalis in a spontaneously conceived singleton pregnancy. *Ultrasound Obstet Gynecol.* 2009;33:371-373.

Suzuki S. Comparison between spontaneous ovarian hyperstimulation syndrome and hyperreactio luteinalis. *Arch Gynecol Obstet.* 2004;269:227-229.

Tube Carcinoma, Primary Fallopian

Synonyms/Description
Tubal carcinoma/malignancy

Etiology
Primary fallopian tube carcinoma (PFTC) is among the rarest gynecologic malignancies, accounting for 0.3% of all gynecologic cancers, and is usually seen in postmenopausal women. There is recent evidence that the majority of high-grade, papillary serous cancers involving the ovary may actually originate in the fallopian tube, then spread to the ovary. There is a precursor lesion of the fallopian tube called serous intraepithelial tubal carcinoma (STIC) that is similar to high-grade ovarian serous adenocarcinoma. Recent research suggests that many ovarian cancers originate from a STIC in the fimbriated end of the fallopian tube. Histologically, up to 90% of tubal cancers are adenocarcinomas, most of which are serous adenocarcinomas. A minority of cases are endometrioid and clear cell adenocarcinoma. The risk factors for tubal cancer are similar to ovarian, including the inheritance of the BRCA 1 and BRCA 2 gene mutations. Approximately 15% to 45% of women with fallopian tube cancer are positive for one of these two mutations. Although the symptoms are nonspecific and may include pain and bleeding, tubal cancer has historically been associated with a characteristic watery vaginal discharge. The Latzko triad includes serosanguineous discharge, colicky pelvic pain, and a mass. Although this triad of symptoms is considered characteristic of tubal cancers, it occurs in only 15% of affected patients.

Ultrasound Findings
The sonographic appearance of tubal carcinoma is very similar to ovarian cancer. There is usually a complex but largely solid adnexal mass with cystic components and abundant blood flow. The mass may be sausage-shaped, suggesting that it may be tubal, but in most cases the ovary is not seen separately. Although hydrosalpinges have a characteristic appearance of incomplete septa and a spoke-wheel pattern, tubal cancers typically have a large solid component obscuring any distinctive features of the tube. Most patients with tubal cancer are presumed preoperatively to have an ovarian malignancy; thus it is rare to make the correct diagnosis prospectively. In a study by Slanetz and colleagues, only 3 of 20 patients were correctly diagnosed sonographically with primary tubal cancer, whereas the others were presumed to be of ovarian origin. These authors also report that the fallopian tube can be a site for metastatic disease from distant primaries.

Differential Diagnosis
The differential diagnosis for tubal cancer is similar to the one for ovarian cancer. The sonographic finding of a complex solid and cystic mass with abundant color flow Doppler and shaggy borders suggests a malignancy. Whether the mass is a tubal, ovarian, or metastatic tumor is indeterminate sonographically. Rarely, there are benign masses that can mimic a tubal or ovarian cancer, such as cystadenofibromas or cystadenomas, with small solid excrescences that may suggest a malignancy. There can also be unusual-appearing degenerating fibroids or complex endometriomas with irregular borders that occasionally simulate a cancer. Generally, tubal cancers tend to be large, multilocular, partly solid, and vascular when discovered, making the diagnosis of a malignancy likely.

Clinical Aspects and Recommendations
The treatment of tubal cancer is similar to the treatment of ovarian cancer. This typically includes surgical debulking by a gynecologic oncologist and referral for medical treatments guided by specialized oncologists.

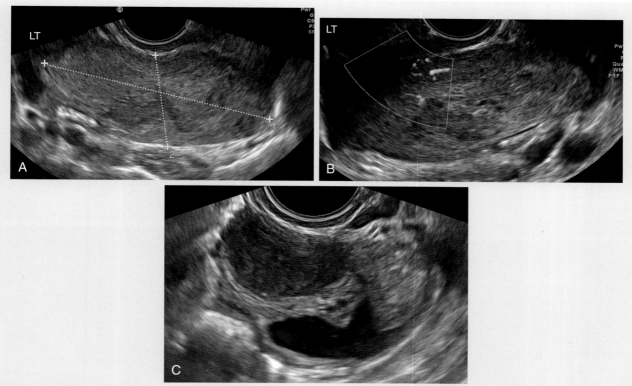

Figure T4-1 Three views of a large tubal carcinoma. **A and B** show the tubular or sausage shape of the solid mass and the prominent vascularity within. **C** is an image taken from the distal end of the same mass, showing several cystic components typical of the complex appearance of tubal cancers.

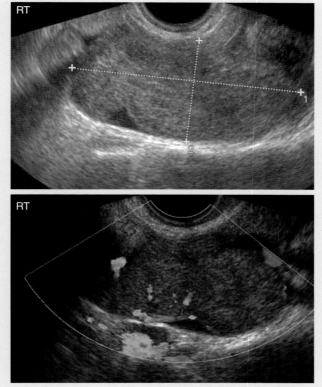

Figure T4-2 Large papillary serous carcinoma of the fallopian tube showing the sausage shape of the solid mass and abundant internal vascularity. This tumor had little if any cystic component.

T

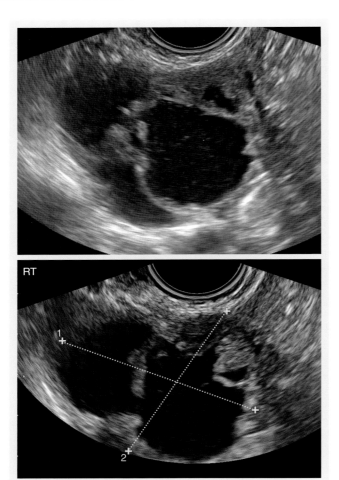

Figure T4-3 Two views of a tubal adenocarcinoma that is predominantly cystic, with thick septa, a thick wall, and areas of internal nodularity. The appearance of this mass is indistinguishable from an ovarian cancer but was proved tubal at surgery.

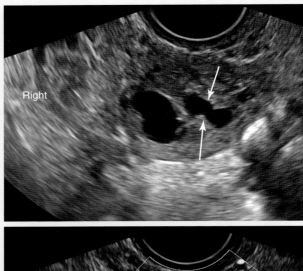

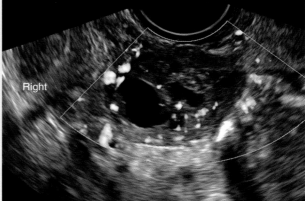

Figure T4-4 Small complex adnexal mass in a postmenopausal patient. The appearance of a solid mass with cystic spaces is nonspecific but consistent with a malignancy. This tubal carcinoma contains a small tubular cystic space *(arrows)* suggesting its tubal origin (only appreciated in retrospect).

Suggested Reading

Chan A, Gilks B, Kwon J, Tinker AV. New insights into the pathogenesis of ovarian carcinoma: time to rethink ovarian cancer screening. *Obstet Gynecol.* 2012;120:935-940.

Haratz-Rubinstein N, Russell B, Gal D. Sonographic diagnosis of fallopian tube carcinoma. *Ultrasound Obstet Gynecol.* 2004;24:86-88.

Huang WC, Yang SH, Yang JM. Ultrasonographic manifestations of fallopian tube carcinoma in the fimbriated end. *J Ultrasound Med.* 2005;24:1157-1160.

Ko ML, Jeng CJ, Chen SC, Tzeng CR. Sonographic appearance of fallopian tube carcinoma. *J Clin Ultrasound.* 2005;33:372-374.

Seidman JD, Zhao P, Yemelyanova A. "Primary peritoneal" high-grade serous carcinoma is very likely metastatic from serous tubal intraepithelial carcinoma: assessing the new paradigm of ovarian and pelvic serous carcinogenesis and its implications for screening for ovarian cancer. *Gynecol Oncol.* 2011;120:470-473.

Slanetz PJ, Whitman GJ, Halpern EF, Hall DA, McCarthy KA, Simeone JF. Imaging of fallopian tube tumors. *Am J Roentgenol.* 1997;169:1321-1324.

Tubo-Ovarian Abcess and Pelvic Inflammatory Disease

Synonyms/Description
Pelvic infection
Pelvic abcess
Pyosalpinx

Etiology
Pelvic inflammatory disease (PID) is an ascending pelvic infection causing inflammation of the upper genital tract, including cervicitis, endometritis, salpingitis, pelvic peritonitis, and occasionally resulting in development of a tubo-ovarian abscess (TOA). Inflammation damages the fallopian tubes, leading to infertility, ectopic pregnancy, and chronic pelvic pain. Acutely, the fallopian tubes swell and become congested, leading to salpingitis and potentially pyosalpinx if the tube fills with pus. Untreated PID may progress from inflammation of the tubo-ovarian complex to the formation of a tubo-ovarian abscess (TOA).

Most cases of PID are sexually transmitted and caused by *Chlamydia trachomatis*, *Neisseria gonorrhoeae*, or other similar causative agents. Pelvic inflammatory disease can also occur as a result of a gynecologic or abdominal procedure or surgery, as well as tuberculosis and appendicitis.

Ultrasound Findings
Ultrasound is very sensitive for detecting ovarian and tubal involvement of PID (sensitivity of 90% and 93%, respectively). When infected, the uterus enlarges and the echogenicity of the endometrium becomes heterogeneous and blotchy. The endometrial cavity often contains small amounts of echogenic fluid (exudate). The outer border of the uterus is often indistinct, with loss of clear separation between the uterus and adnexa.

Inflamed fallopian tubes are typically thick walled and dilated, filled with echogenic fluid and debris. The walls are irregular, and the tubes are elongated and tortuous with abundant blood flow on color Doppler examination. Milder infections may result in thickening of the tube without the presence of fluid (salpingitis). These thickened tubes are very tender during the transvaginal ultrasound examination.

A TOA is usually a solid, cystic or complex multiseptate mass, most often hypoechoic with areas of mixed echogenicity and thick septa.

Adhesions form within the pelvis, causing the tubo-ovarian complex to be adherent to nearby bowel, giving the appearance of a large, complex, adnexal mass with indistinct borders. Abundant blood flow is typical on Doppler studies.

Differential Diagnosis
The sonographic appearance of PID and TOA is nonspecific, and the differential diagnosis includes diseases that can cause complex hydrosalpinges and pain. These include ectopic pregnancy (there must be a positive pregnancy test), extensive endometriosis (typically a patient with chronic, cyclic pelvic pain), and tubal carcinoma (typically asymptomatic). Patients with PID and TOA are usually febrile and appear quite ill; therefore the clinical setting is an important part of evaluating a patient with a complex multiseptate tubo-ovarian mass.

Clinical Aspects and Recommendations
PID and TOAs are infections of the upper reproductive tract, usually sexually transmitted but occasionally polymicrobial; therefore, treatment is with antibiotics. The choice of antibiotics depends on the source of infection. The diagnosis of PID is more of a clinical diagnosis than one based on ultrasound findings. Clinicians are taught to maintain a low threshold for suspecting,

T

diagnosing, and treating PID because long-term complications are more common if treatment is delayed. Easily obtainable sensitive pregnancy tests have helped quickly exclude possible ectopic pregnancy in patients who present with lower abdominal pain. Appendicitis and ovarian torsion are part of a clinical differential and may be assisted by ultrasound findings. TOAs may be more chronic and the diagnosis better assisted by the presence of complex adnexal masses as well as clinical signs, symptoms, and laboratory findings. Antibiotics or surgical intervention may be indicated, but specific recommendations are beyond the scope of this book.

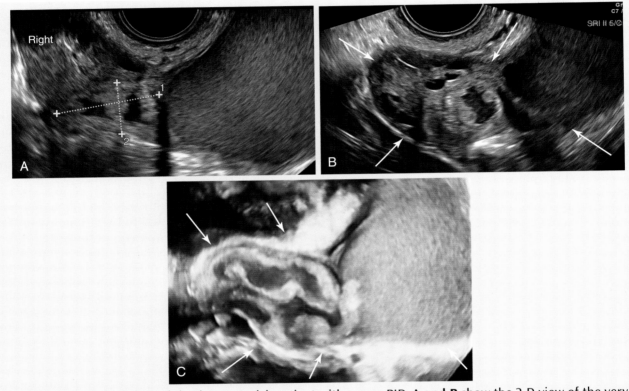

Figure T5-1   Very large pyosalpinx in a very sick patient with severe PID. **A and B** show the 2-D view of the very large pyosalpinx. The distal end of the tube is filled with a large amount of echogenic fluid. The rest of tube is more narrow and folded upon itself *(calipers and arrows)*. **C** is a 3-D rendering of the entire dilated tube *(arrows)*.

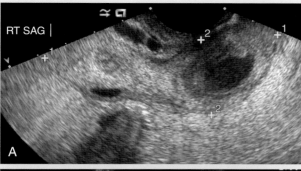

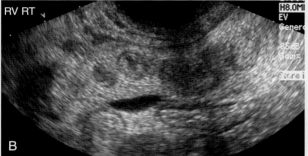

Figure T5-2   A and B, Acute PID with a very dilated tube in a patient later found to have a TOA. Note that the tubal wall is thick and edematous with multiple cystic spaces (pockets of pus) inside.

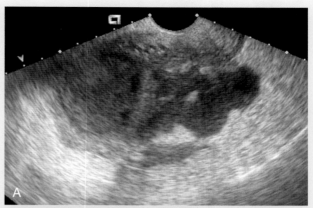

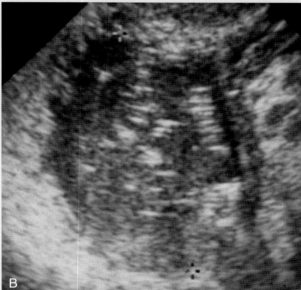

Figure T5-3   Tubo-ovarian abscess in two different patients. A shows a large complex cystic mass with irregular borders and septations in a patient with severe PID. Note that the borders of the mass are indistinct and blurry because of the surrounding edema. Although the sonographic appearance of the mass is nonspecific, the setting of a septic patient helps to make the diagnosis more definitive. **B** shows a completely solid adnexal mass containing small linear echoes throughout, consistent with an air-containing abscess.

T

T

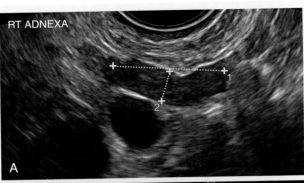

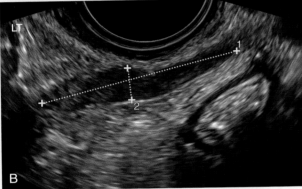

Figure T5-4   A and B, Salpingitis in two different patients. Note the elongated and straight swollen-appearing tubes *(calipers)*. Both patients had localized pain in the area of the tube. For the patient in **A,** the diagnosis of pyosalpinx was confirmed at laparoscopy. The second patient improved with antibiotics.

Suggested Reading

Chappell CA, Wiesenfeld HC. Pathogenesis, diagnosis, and management of severe pelvic inflammatory disease and tuboovarian abscess. *Clin Obstet Gynecol.* 2012;55:893-903.

Cicchiello LA, Hamper UM, Scoutt LM. Ultrasound evaluation of gynecologic causes of pelvic pain. *Obstet Gynecol Clin North Am.* 2011;38:85-114.

Crossman SH. The challenge of pelvic inflammatory disease. *Am Fam Physician.* 2006;73:859-864.

Ghiatas AA. The spectrum of pelvic inflammatory disease. *Eur Radiol.* 2004;14(suppl):E184-E192.

Kamaya A, Shin L, Chen B, Desser TS. Emergency gynecologic imaging. *Semin Ultrasound CT MRI.* 2008;29:353-368.

Kim MY, Rha SE, Oh SN, Jung SE, Lee YJ, Kim YS, Byun JY, Lee A, Kim MR. MR imaging findings of hydrosalpinx: a comprehensive review. *Radiographics.* 2009;29:495-507.

Soper DE. Pelvic inflammatory disease. *Obstet Gynecol.* 2010;116:419-428.

Varras M, Polyzos D, Perouli E, Noti P, Pantazis I, Akrivis CH. Tubo-ovarian abscesses: spectrum of sonographic findings with surgical and pathological correlations. *Clin Exp Obstet Gynecol.* 2003;30:117-121.

Ureteral Stone

Synonyms/Description
Renal stone
Kidney stone
Nephrolithiasis

Etiology
Renal and ureteral stones are typically calcium stones (calcium oxalate, calcium phosphate, or mixed calcium oxalate and phosphate). A minority (20%) of stones are uric acid, cystine, and struvite in origin. They become especially symptomatic when they travel down the ureter and become lodged, causing a blockage in the flow of urine.

Ultrasound Findings
Sonography is very useful in visualizing stones at the ureteropelvic junction (UPJ), the ureterovesical junction (UVJ), the renal pelvis, and in the kidney itself, although stones are harder to see when located in the mid ureter. Patlas and colleagues reported a sensitivity and specificity of 95% and 93%, respectively, for diagnosing ureteral calculi, although unfortunately a majority of urologists are still ordering CT scans for the workup of renal colic. Stones lodged in the distal ureter are easily seen sonographically either transabdominally through a full bladder, or even better transvaginally. Ureteral calculi are echogenic foci with acoustic shadowing, seen within the lumen of a dilated ureter. There is usually associated ipsilateral hydronephrosis and flank pain. Partial obstruction of the distal ureter may also cause asymmetry of the ureteral jets in the bladder (seen best using color Doppler in the urinary bladder).

Differential Diagnosis
Patients with flank pain who are scheduled for pelvic ultrasound should also have a cursory examination of the ipsilateral kidney. If there is evidence of hydronephrosis, the ultrasound examination should include a careful look at the course of the ureter, including the junction of the distal ureter and the bladder, which is best done transvaginally. If there is a stone at the UVJ, there is essentially no differential diagnosis. Occasionally there may be other disease processes in that location, such as a bladder mass or endometriosis, causing constriction of the distal ureter and mimicking the symptoms of a stone (see Bladder Masses).

Clinical Aspects and Recommendations
Patients with ureteral stones have extreme, crampy flank pain, with tenderness at the costovertebral angle (CVA). Most patients (90%) have gross or microscopic hematuria. The treatment for ureteral stones requires referral to a urologist, who may remove or break up (i.e., lithotripsy) the stone if spontaneous passage does not occur.

U

U

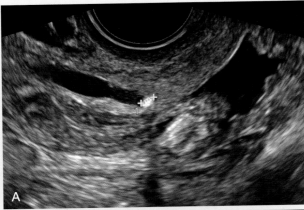

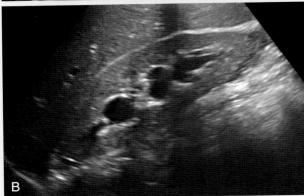

Suggested Reading

Ackerman SJ, Irshad A, Anis M. Ultrasound for pelvic pain II: nongynecologic causes. *Obstet Gynecol Clin North Am.* 2011;38:69-83.

Masarani M, Dinneen M. Ureteric colic: new trends in diagnosis and treatment. *Postgrad Med J.* 2007;83: 469-472. Review.

Patlas M, Farkas A, Fisher D, Zaghal I, Hadas-Halpern I. Ultrasound vs CT for the detection of ureteric stones in patients with renal colic. *Br J Radiol.* 2001;74:901-904.

Figure U1-1 **A** shows a stone *(calipers)* lodged in the distal ureter of a patient with flank pain. Note that the stone has a posterior acoustic shadow and is located at the distal end of the dilated, fluid-containing ureter. **B** shows the kidney on the ipsilateral side with moderate hydronephrosis.

Uterine Sarcoma

Synonyms/Description

Many different types of uterine sarcoma, including but not limited to carcinosarcoma, adenosarcoma, leiomyosarcoma, and endometrial stromal sarcoma

Etiology

Uterine sarcomas are rare tumors of mesenchymal origin, representing approximately 5% of all uterine malignancies.

They are classified into three groups according to their source:

1. Mixed epithelial and mesenchymal tumors, which include carcinosarcomas. These were previously termed malignant mixed Müllerian tumors (MMMTs) and adenosarcomas.
2. Smooth muscle tumors, which are leiomyosarcomas
3. Endometrial stromal tumors, which include endometrial stromal sarcoma and high-grade undifferentiated sarcoma

Carcinosarcoma is the most common, accounting for 50% of all uterine sarcomas. It is typically diagnosed in the sixth decade and often presents with postmenopausal bleeding. The presentation and risk factors are similar to endometrial adenocarcinoma. It is an aggressive tumor with extrauterine spread to lymph nodes or beyond found in 30% of patients at initial diagnosis.

Adenosarcoma is a less aggressive tumor than carcinosarcoma. It tends to be smaller and confined to the uterus at presentation and has a more favorable prognosis.

Leiomyosarcoma is the second most common uterine sarcoma, occurs mostly in the fifth decade of life, and accounts for almost 40% of cases. These tumors are not thought to arise from existing myomas. They generally present with the same symptoms attributed to enlarging fibroids and rapid growth of the uterus.

Endometrial stromal sarcomas represent approximately 10% of uterine sarcomas and typically present with vaginal bleeding and pelvic pain in women 40 to 55 years of age.

Ultrasound Findings

Uterine sarcomas usually present as large uterine masses that may be difficult to distinguish from fibroids. They can be polypoid with cystic spaces and ill-defined borders. They often involve the endometrium, at least in part, and may prolapse or extend through the endocervical canal. This type may be mistaken for a submucosal degenerating fibroid or an endometrial polyp. The appearance of a vascular, intraluminal mass can also mimic endometrial adenocarcinoma. Doppler usually shows abundant blood flow as is common in malignancies. The diagnosis of a sarcoma may be suspected if the mass is irregular with disorganized cystic areas and especially if the mass is rapidly growing and very vascular. Leiomyosarcomas are typically difficult to distinguish from highly vascular benign leiomyomas by imaging alone.

Differential Diagnosis

The differential diagnosis for a large uterine mass with irregular cystic areas includes a degenerating fibroid and an adenomyoma. These typically do not grow and do not have the abundant blood flow seen in a sarcoma. Endometrial cancers can also grow to a large size and look like a sarcoma; however, endometrial cancers are typically less aggressive and usually present at an earlier stage with abnormal bleeding. Because fibroids are far more common than sarcomas, a uterine mass may be mistaken for an atypical fibroid at first scan. If a fibroid is unusual in appearance, it is important to rescan the patient in a relatively short time interval to evaluate growth of the lesion.

U

Clinical Aspects and Recommendations

Five-year overall survival for patients with stage 1 to 2 uterine carcinosarcoma is 44% to 74%. The survival for women with stage 1 to 2 leiomyosarcoma is 52% to 85%.

Endometrial stromal sarcoma has the best prognosis, with a 90% 5-year survival rate in women with stage I disease. Survival is poor in patients with stage III to IV disease for all types of sarcomas.

The treatment for uterine sarcomas depends on the type of tumor and the extent of disease. Uterine sarcomas are relatively rare and should be managed at specialized centers because treatments are typically multimodal and evolving. Recurrence rates are relatively high compared with other types of gynecologic malignancies.

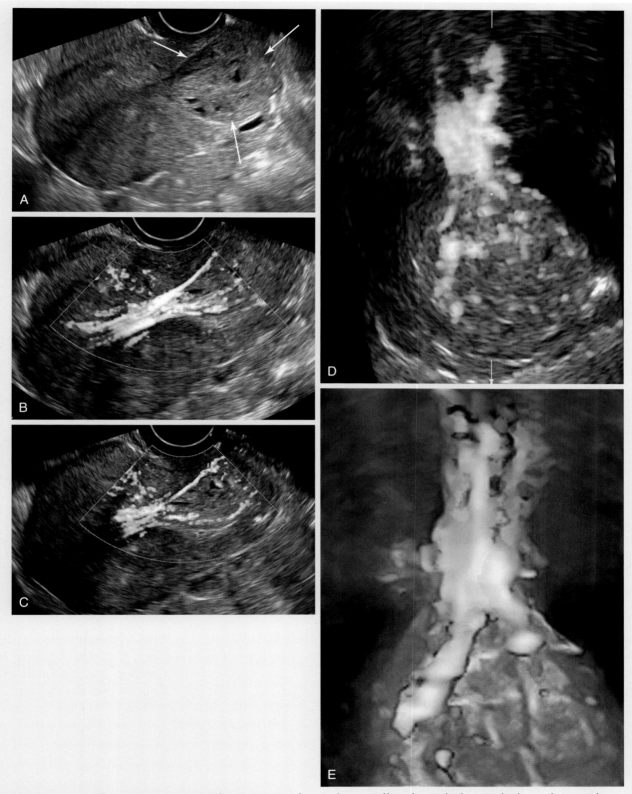

Figure U2-1   A, Adenosarcoma presenting as a mass *(arrows)* protruding through the cervical canal. Note the small cystic areas within the solid matrix of the mass. **B and C** show abundant color flow with a large stalk originating from the uterine fundus. **D and E** show a 3-D image of the vasculature of the mass as it attempts to pass through the cervix.

U

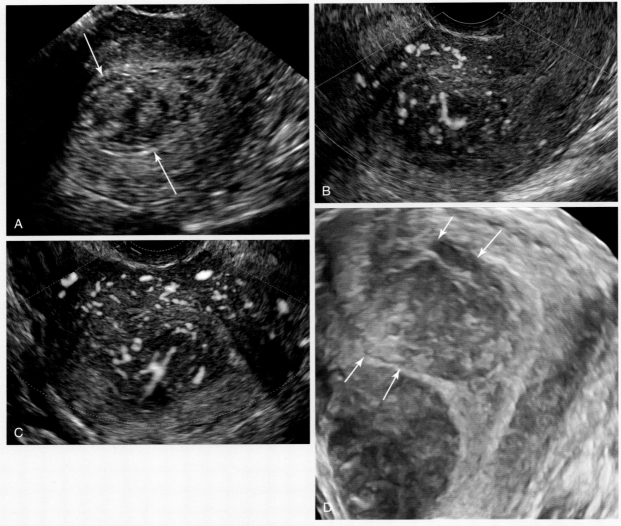

Figure U2-2 Endometrial stromal sarcoma. **A,** Note that the solid mass *(arrows)* is largely intraluminal; however, the color flow images **(B and C)** show abundant blood flow coming from the uterine fundus where the borders of the mass are ill-defined. **D** is a 3-D rendered image of the endometrial cavity showing a sharp border on one side but no real border *(arrows)* at the right fundus where the tumor appears to reach the serosa.

Suggested Reading

Seddon BM, Davda R. Uterine sarcomas—recent progress and future challenges. *Eur J Radiol.* 2011; 78(1):30-40.

Shah SH, Jagannathan JP, Krajewski K, O'Regan KN, George S, Ramaiya NH. Uterine sarcomas: then and now. *AJR Am J Roentgenol.* 2012;199(1):213-223.

Wu TI, Yen TC, Lai CH. Clinical presentation and diagnosis of uterine sarcoma, including imaging. *Best Pract Res Clin Obstet Gynaecol.* 2011;25(6):681-689.

Xue WC, Cheung AN. Endometrial stromal sarcoma of uterus. *Best Pract Res Clin Obstet Gynaecol.* 2011;25(6):719-732.

Vaginal Masses

Synonyms/Description
None

Etiology
The most common vaginal masses are benign.

Vaginal Cysts
Vaginal wall cysts tend to be embryologic in nature and often asymptomatic. These cysts include Gartner's duct cysts, Müllerian cysts, epithelial inclusion cysts (ectopic epithelium), urethral diverticula, and cysts resulting from a blocked gland Bartholin duct cyst) or obstructed Müllerian duct anomaly. A complete vaginal septum will typically be diagnosed during menarche when a hematometra develops from the obstructed menstrual flow (see Hematometra and Hematocolpos). Gartner's duct cysts are remnants of the mesonephric ducts and are most often discovered incidentally. They are located along the anterolateral aspect of the vagina and are typically clear unilocular cysts. Bartholin's glands are mucus-secreting glands in the posterolateral aspect of the vaginal opening, near the rectum. Bartholin's duct cysts result from blockage of the duct and swelling from accumulated secretions.

Kondi-Pafiti and colleagues studied 40 cases of benign vaginal cysts. Of these, 12 cases were Müllerian cysts (30.0%), 11 were Bartholin's duct cysts (27.5%), 10 were epidermal inclusion cysts (25.0%), 5 were Gartner's duct cysts (12.5%), 1 was an endometrioid cyst (2.5%), and 1 was an unclassified cyst (2.5%). Mean patient age was 35 years (range 20 to 75). Most of the patients (31 cases, 77.5%) were asymptomatic, and the Bartholin's duct cyst was the more frequently symptomatic.

Vaginal Solid Masses
Fibroids may occur in the vagina, originating from the smooth muscle cells of the anterior vagina or vesicovaginal septum. These are usually solid rounded masses that are well encapsulated and not particularly vascular. Implants of endometriosis are commonly found in the rectovaginal septum or along the posterior wall of the bladder, and may indent or involve the vaginal wall. Malignant masses in the vagina are very rare. Metastatic spread (such as lymphoma or melanoma) accounts for the most common malignant masses in the vagina, followed by primary squamous cell carcinoma. Primary vaginal cancers represent only 1% to 2% of all gynecologic malignancies, and 85% of these primary vaginal malignancies are squamous cell carcinoma. Other rare primary vaginal cancers include adenocarcinoma, melanoma, lymphoma, and sarcomas.

Postoperative or radiation changes may result in vaginal lesions secondary to inflammation and fibrosis. Fistulas between the vagina and rectum can present with vaginal symptoms.

Ultrasound Findings
The best way to evaluate the vagina sonographically is by placing a high-frequency transducer (such as the transvaginal probe) on the perineum and by looking down the vagina, rectum, and urethra simultaneously. Once the vaginal probe is actually inserted into the vagina, it will bypass any vaginal pathology, and the vaginal findings will be obscured and undetectable.

A 3-D acquisition taken from the perineum is important to generate the coronal view of the floor of the pelvis. Using that reconstructed view, the vagina, urethra, and rectum can be seen in cross-section and their relationship with one another evaluated. This view can demonstrate the location of the mass within the floor of the pelvis, specifically showing the relationship of the mass to the vagina, urethra, and rectum. This reconstructed view of the pelvic floor is also ideal to demonstrate defects in the vaginal wall such as fistulas (see Figure V1-9), and is increasingly being used in urogynecology. Similar to any other pelvic mass, the appearance of the vaginal mass, such as gray-scale texture, contour, and degree of vascularity using color flow Doppler, provides clues as to the diagnosis. The location of the mass is also important, keeping in mind that masses in the anterior compartment may be urologic and those in the posterior compartment may be gastrointestinal. The vagina, urethra, and rectum are in close proximity to one another, sharing walls that may be affected by the mass. Refer to the differential diagnosis section that follows for a description and comparison of these masses and their sonographic appearance.

Differential Diagnosis

A clear and asymptomatic cyst in the lateral wall of the vagina is likely to be a Gartner's duct cyst. Fluid (or blood) in a hemi-hematocolpos secondary to a vaginal septum typically has low-level echoes indicating unclotted blood, much like an ovarian endometrioma. A complex cyst with solid elements seen anterior to the vagina suggests a urethral diverticulum. When the lesion is symptomatic, peripheral color flow may be seen, owing to inflammation. A complex cyst in the posterior-lateral wall of the vagina is likely to be a Bartholin's duct cyst and has only peripheral color flow. The most common rounded and focal solid mass (with limited color flow) is a fibroid in the vaginal wall.

Although vaginal cysts are usually benign, most solid vaginal masses with abundant color flow tend to be malignant. The appearance of the solid mass is not useful to determine the specific tissue diagnosis, as sarcomas, lymphomas, and other lesions look similar to one another. Malignant vaginal masses are typically completely solid, abundantly vascular, and irregular in contour. They may extend into the surrounding tissues such as the pelvic side walls.

Clinical Aspects and Recommendations

The treatment of vaginal masses depends on the diagnosis. Benign cysts are treated depending on the patient's symptoms. Asymptomatic Gartner's duct cysts are typically monitored with follow-up ultrasounds, whereas a symptomatic Bartholin's duct cyst requires drainage or marsupialization. Urethral diverticula may be found incidentally or when they become symptomatic, and are usually managed by a urogynecologist or urologist. Treatment of malignant vaginal masses depends on the specific type of malignancy and usually involves a multidisciplinary team including gynecologic and medical oncology.

V

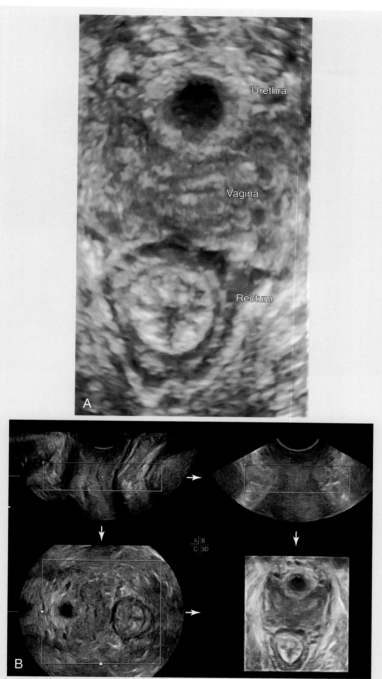

Figure V1-1   A and B, 3-D reconstructed view of the floor of the normal pelvis, showing the urethra, vagina, and rectum en face. **B** demonstrates the multiplanar view of the pelvic floor, showing the acquisition planes. The 3-D volume was acquired from the perineum and sweeping side to side. The A plane in the upper left-hand corner shows the acquisition view looking straight down the vagina. The B plane shows the same view at right angles from the A plane. The C plane is the reconstructed view of the floor of the pelvis, which is crucial to evaluating the perineal structures, including the length of the vagina and its relationship to neighboring structures.

V

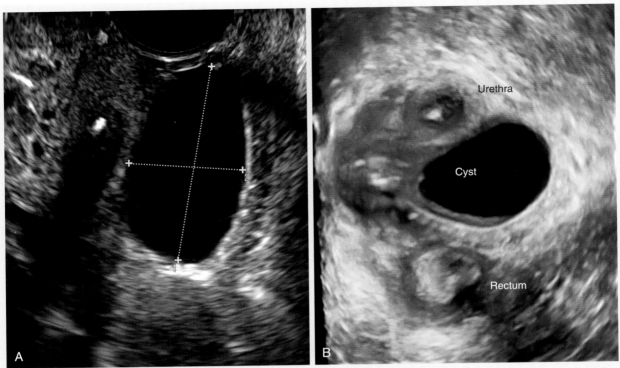

Figure V1-2   A and B, Gartner's duct cyst: Long axis view looking down the vagina from the perineum, showing a clear unilocular cyst just posterior to the urethra. **B** is a 3-D reconstructed image of the pelvic floor, showing that the cyst is located along the left side of the vagina.

V

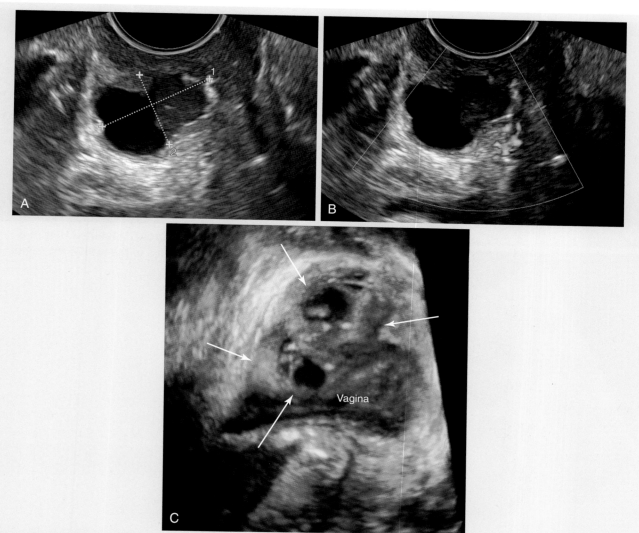

Figure V1-3 Urethral diverticulum. **A and B,** 2-D view of a complex cystic mass with irregular borders and internal debris. Note that the vascularity is only in the peripheral aspect of the mass. The mass was located anterior to the vagina and lateral to the urethra. The patient was quite symptomatic, particularly upon voiding. **C,** 3-D reconstructed view of a different case of a urethral diverticulum. Note the complex, multicystic mass anterior to the vagina where the urethra should be. The exact location of the urethra is obscured and likely encapsulated by this cystic mass, which was quite symptomatic.

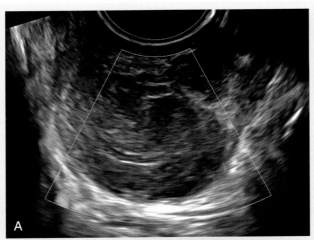

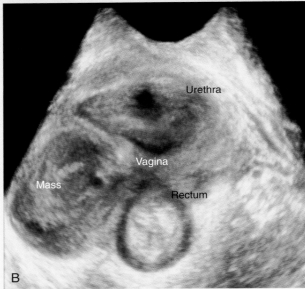

Figure V1-4 Bartholin's duct cyst. **(A)** 2-D and **(B)** 3-D views of a heterogeneous solid mass located antero-lateral to the rectum. Note that the interior of the mass has no discernible blood flow.

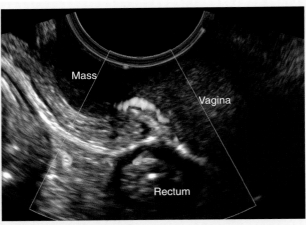

Figure V1-5 Vaginal fibroid. Magnified view of a small, rounded, solid mass in the wall of the vagina.

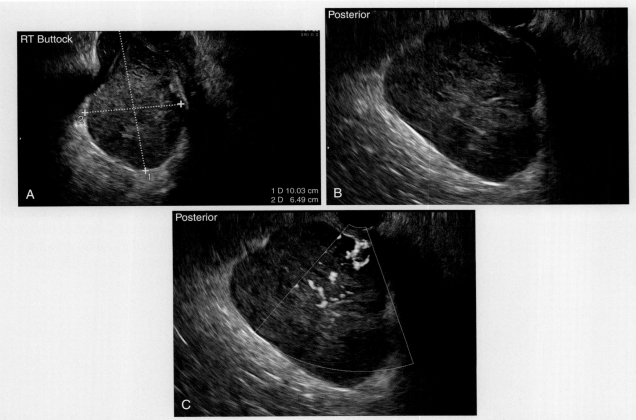

Figure V1-6   A to C, Leiomyosarcoma. Multiple views of a solid and very vascular mass located along the right side of the vagina and extending posteriorly toward the right buttock.

V

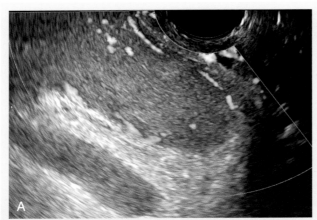

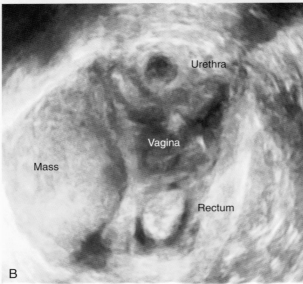

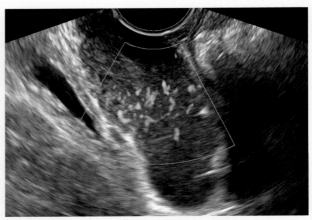

Figure V1-8 Vaginal lymphoma. Long axis view from the perineum, looking down the vagina, showing a lobulated irregular vascular mass extending the entire length of the vagina.

Figure V1-7 **A and B,** Myxoid spindle cell sarcoma. Very vascular, lobulated and irregular solid mass along the lateral and posterior aspect of the vagina. Note that the mass has a fingerlike extension into the surrounding side wall, indicating the aggressive behavior of the tumor.

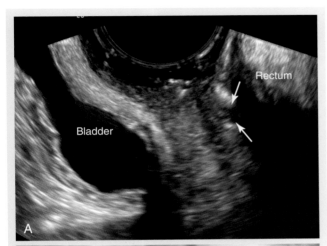

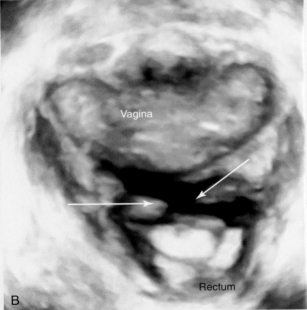

Figure V1-9 **A and B,** Recto-vaginal fistula. 2-D and 3-D views of the perineum looking down the vagina in a patient with Crohn's disease who had clinical evidence of a fistula. Arrows demonstrate the location of the fistula, which was identified first on the 3-D reconstruction (**B**) and then recognized on standard 2-D imaging (**A**). An MRI done the same day had been read as negative.

Suggested Reading

Dai Y, Wang J, Shen H, Zhao RN, Li YZ. Diagnosis of female urethral diverticulum using transvaginal contrast-enhanced sonourethrography. *J Int Urogynecol*. January 31, 2013. [Epub ahead of print].

Elsayes KM, Narra VR, Dillman JR, Velcheti V, Hameed O, Tongdee R, Menias CO. Vaginal masses: magnetic resonance imaging features with pathologic correlation. *Acta Radiol*. 2007;48:921-933.

Fletcher SG, Lemack GE. Benign masses of the female periurethral tissues and anterior vaginal wall. *Curr Urol Rep*. 2008;9:389-396.

Hwang JH, Oh JM, Lee NW, Hur JY, Lee KW, Lee KJ. Multiple vaginal Müllerian cysts: a case report and review of literature. *Arch Gynecol Obstet*. 2009;280:137-139.

Kondi-Pafiti A, Grapsa D, Papakonstantinou K, Kairi-Vassilatou E, Xasiakos D. Vaginal cysts: a common pathologic entity revisited. *Clin Exp Obstet Gynecol*. 2008;35:41-44.

Normal Pelvic Ultrasound and Common Normal Variants

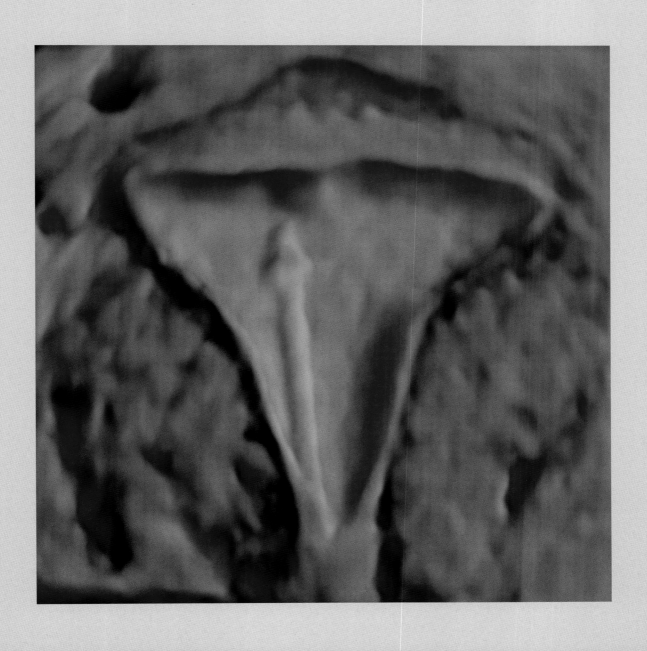

Normal Pelvic Ultrasound and Common Normal Variants

The Normal Pelvic Ultrasound: How to Do It and What to See

Knowledge of the normal anatomy and techniques for scanning the female pelvis are essential for detecting pelvic disease. The complete pelvic sonogram is done in two parts. In most cases, these include the transabdominal followed by the transvaginal evaluation. Decades ago, the transabdominal pelvic ultrasound was performed using a full bladder to visualize the pelvic organs by pushing the bowel out of the way. Although on occasion filling the patient's bladder may be helpful, the transabdominal scan is very effective even if the bladder is not completely distended. If the uterus is anteverted, it is typically well seen whether or not the bladder is full. A retroverted uterus may be difficult to visualize with an empty bladder; however, it will be seen well transvaginally. Hence it is no longer necessary to obligate patients to fill their bladders for pelvic ultrasound, assuming that the transvaginal scan is also performed. If for some reason the patient is to be scanned with a full bladder (e.g., if the patient declines the intravaginal scan), it is important not to overdistend the bladder, thus compressing the pelvic organs against the sacrum.

The pelvic scan should typically include a transvaginal component after the transabdominal scan unless contraindicated or declined by the patient. If the patient is not a candidate for the transvaginal approach, the scan can be performed transrectally (see technique that follows).

The technique for performing a transabdominal (TA) scan (Figure II-1):

1. The uterus is imaged both longitudinally and transversely using a 3- to 8-MHz abdominal transducer. If the bladder is full, it can be used as an acoustic window because it lies just anterior to the uterus. If the bladder is not distended, gentle pressure can be applied to the abdominal wall with the transducer to push the bowel away and narrow the distance between the probe and the pelvic organs. If the uterus is large or contains fibroids, the TA approach may provide the best view and measurements of the uterus. This perspective may even improve after the bladder is emptied. It is important to image the endometrial lining as well as ensure that the fundus of the uterus has been fully imaged. Looking just above the uterus is often necessary to detect any masses in the lower abdomen, when they are too cephalad to be visualized transvaginally.

2. The adnexa are evaluated, providing slight pressure on the lower abdominal organs to improve visibility. This gentle pressure can displace the bowel and better visualize the adnexal regions. The ovaries themselves may not be identified until the transvaginal portion of the scan; however, the overall evaluation of the right and left lower quadrants often requires a TA view in patients in whom there an ovary or mass located high in the pelvis or lower abdomen.

The technique for performing the transvaginal (TV) scan (Figure II-2):

1. Proper disinfection of the transvaginal probe is essential preceding each use, and should be performed in accordance with the standard guidelines recommended by each institution (hospital) or probe manufacturer. Following disinfection, the probe is rinsed with water to remove any residual chemicals and wiped clean. It is then inserted into a probe cover that typically contains coupling gel. Finally the tip of the probe is lubricated before its insertion into the vagina. If the scan is being

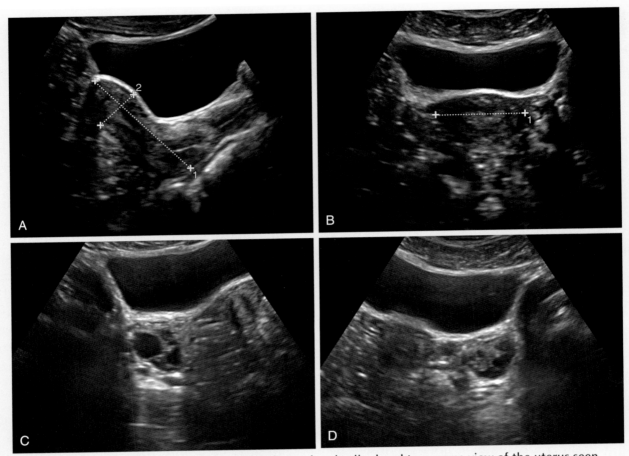

Figure II-1   Transabdominal scan (TA). **A and B** show a longitudinal and transverse view of the uterus seen transabdominally through a distended bladder. Calipers show the measurements of the uterus. **C and D** show the normal ovaries, also seen transabdominally.

done for infertility and the patient is a candidate for insemination, it is crucial not to use a gel that may be harmful to the sperm, and water or saline can be utilized in these special circumstances.

2. The TV scan is typically done with an empty bladder (except for rare instances in which the bladder itself is to be evaluated); therefore, the patient should empty her bladder just before initiating the TV scan.

3. The vaginal probe can be introduced into the vagina by a physician, a sonographer, or the patient herself, whichever is most appropriate and comfortable for the patient. In certain cases, a chaperone may be necessary, especially if the physician or sonographer is male.

The technique for performing the transrectal (TR) scan (Figure II-3):

1. After emptying her bladder, the patient is placed in the Sims position, on her side with her legs tucked toward her abdomen or maintained in a dorsolithotomy position.

2. The transvaginal transducer is prepared in the same way as for TV scan, and inserted into the rectum by the physician or sonographer. The insertion is done very slowly, with steady but gentle pressure, and under direct visualization of the rectum (sonographically), thus giving time for the sphincter to relax. One can also perform a digital rectal exam preceding the probe insertion to relax the sphincter muscle and gauge the

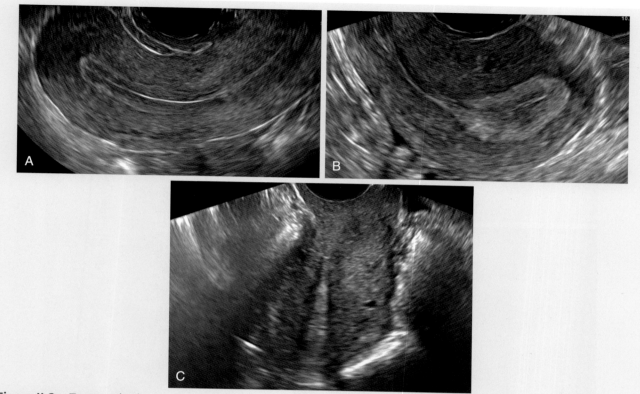

Figure II-2   Transvaginal scan (TV). **A** demonstrates the transvaginal view of a normal anteverted uterus seen longitudinally. **B** shows a similar view of a normal retroverted uterus. Note that in both cases the body of the uterus is at right angles to the ultrasound beam. **C** shows an axial uterus that is hard to image well transvaginally because of its vertical orientation away from the ultrasound beam.

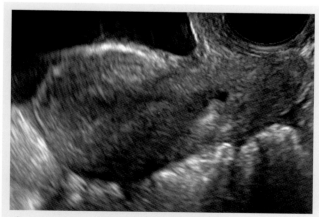

Figure II-3   Transrectal scan. The uterus is seen longitudinally in the same orientation as if the probe were in the vagina. The scan is being done transrectally on a virginal patient.

direction of the rectum. In the Sims position, when the cervix is visualized and approximately half of the shaft of the probe is inside the rectum, the patient is then carefully turned onto her back while trying not to dislodge the probe. With the patient supine, the pelvic landmarks become similar to those seen transvaginally, and the protocol is the same.

Protocol for Intracavitary Scan
The Vagina
To assess the vagina, it is important to visualize the entire length of the vagina from the introitus, before placing the vaginal probe inside (Figure II-4, *A* and *B*). Once the probe is inside the vagina, the vaginal walls and surrounding

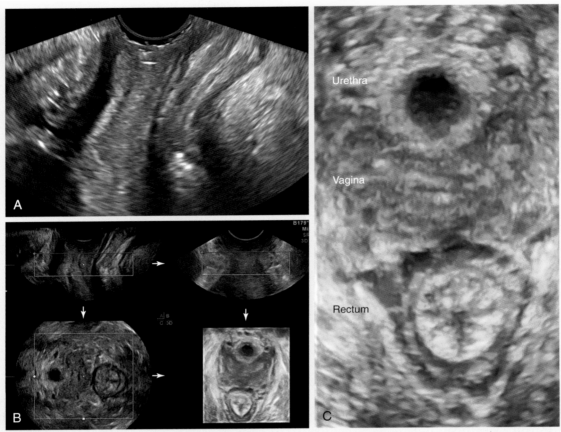

Figure II-4   The perineum. **A** shows a longitudinal scan of the floor of the pelvis looking from the introitus, down the length of the vagina. **B and C** show the 3-D volume acquisition with the axial reconstructed transverse view of the pelvic floor. The reconstructed view shows the urethra, vagina, and rectum in transverse section.

structures are no longer visible. An attempt to visualize them on the way out of the vagina is hampered by the introduction of air with the initial placement of the probe; hence if the clinical problem involves the vagina, it must be evaluated with a perineal scan before placing the probe inside. With the probe on the perineum, a 3-D volume can be acquired and reconstructed to show the floor of the pelvis, the anterior and posterior compartments of the pelvis (Figure II-4, *B* and *C*). This enables the practitioner to assess the relationships between the urethra, vagina, and rectum and any mass or cyst that may be present (see Vaginal Masses).

The Cervix

The appearance, size, and symmetry of the cervix are evaluated as well as the cervical canal

for any polyps, fibroids or masses (Figure II-5). Color Doppler is helpful to detect abnormal blood flow or a feeder vessel if a polyp or mass is suspected. Small cysts in the wall of the cervix are usually nabothian cysts, also referred to as cervical inclusion cysts, and typically are ignored on a sonogram. Evaluating the outer contour of the cervix is important to look for implants of endometriosis along the posterior outer surface of the cervix and in the upper portion of the rectovaginal septum (see Endometriosis).

The Uterus

As the vaginal probe is placed in the vagina, there is direct visualization of the length of the vagina down to the cervix, which is typically at right angles to the vagina (Figures II-2 and II-6).

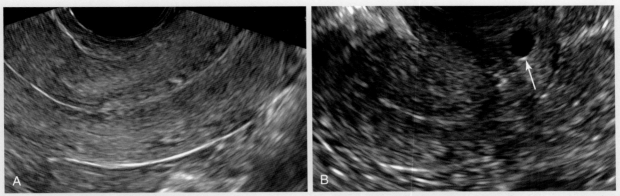

Figure II-5 The cervix. **A** shows a transvaginal longitudinal view of the normal cervix showing a normal endocervical canal. **B** demonstrates a nabothian cyst *(arrow)* located in the cervix of a postmenopausal patient. These are of no clinical significance and typically are not mentioned in the ultrasound report.

Once the cervix is located, the cul-de-sac is seen posteriorly (Figure II-7) and the rest of the uterus is visualized longitudinally. The evaluation of the uterus includes the uterine orientation, location of the endometrium, and symmetry of the myometrium. If the uterus is anteverted or retroverted, it will be seen at right angles (horizontal) to the ultrasound beam and be easily examined (see Figure II-2). If the uterus is axial, it will be oriented parallel and heading away from the ultrasound beam and be much more difficult to image (see Figure II-2). In such cases the endometrial cavity may be better seen TA. The measurements of the uterus that are done longitudinally include the uterine length from the fundus to the cervix (external os), and the width from the anterior to posterior uterine surfaces, perpendicular to the length. The width of the uterus is measured in the transverse view, with the uterus viewed in short axis. These measurements can be done either TA or TV (see Figures II-1 and II-8).

The texture of the myometrium is evaluated for contour changes, heterogeneity, masses, bulges, and cysts. Fibroids or other masses must be measured in at least two dimensions. It is important to determine the location of fibroids within the uterus such as whether it is submucosal, intramural, subserosal or pedunculated (see Fibroids). Postmenopausal women may have extensive calcification of the arcuate arteries, which is not

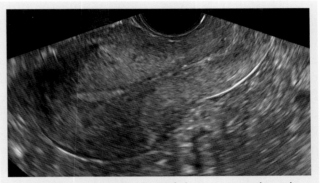

Figure II-6 Long axis view of the uterus and cervix, typical of the first landmark to visualize when performing a vaginal ultrasound.

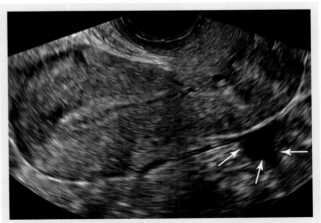

Figure II-7 Longitudinal scan though the uterus and cervix showing a small amount of free fluid *(arrows)* in the cul-de-sac, which is a normal finding, particularly in premenopausal patients.

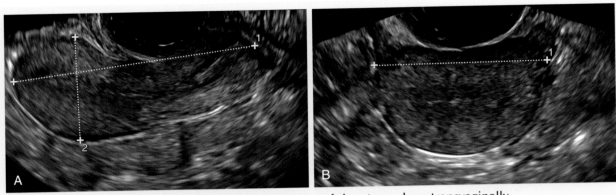

Figure II-8   A and B, Measurements of the uterus done transvaginally.

associated with any gynecological abnormalities (Figure II-9).

The endometrium should be assessed for its appearance, thickness, and focal irregularities or disruptions (Figure II-10). The presence of fluid in the endometrial cavity should be evaluated; if fluid is present, it should be noted whether it outlines any focal or diffuse abnormalities, defects, or masses protruding into the cavity. The endometrium should be measured in the midline on a longitudinal image where the axis of the uterus is perpendicular to the ultrasound beam (Figure II-11). Any rotation of the uterus may artificially widen this measurement; therefore, the axis of the probe should mimic the axis of the uterus. If there is fluid in the endometrial cavity, the endometrial measurement can be obtained by measuring the single width anterior and posterior portions of the endometrium separately. A small amount of anechoic fluid is not considered to be an abnormal finding, and is more commonly seen in postmenopausal patients. Regardless of what the endometrial echo measures, it is essential to evaluate the endometrium in its entirety, looking for focal abnormalities or irregularities. The endometrial echo may be normal on one side of the uterus and have a focal lesion on the other. When finding an endometrial abnormality, color Doppler can

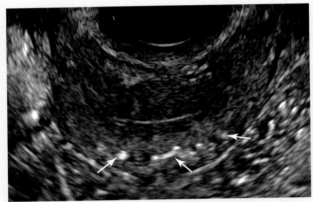

Figure II-9   Transverse view of the uterus in a postmenopausal patient who has multiple arcuate artery calcifications *(arrows)*. These are not considered of clinical significance.

be very helpful to further delineate the lesion (see Figure II-11, C).

The appearance of the endometrium varies with the phases of the menstrual cycle. In the early proliferative phase, it is very thin, echogenic, and linear (Figure II-12). During the proliferative phase, the endometrium gradually thickens. Closer to the time of ovulation (midcycle), the endometrium typically develops a characteristic trilaminar appearance with a thin linear echogenic line at the center, flanked by an echolucent rim and surrounded by an echogenic

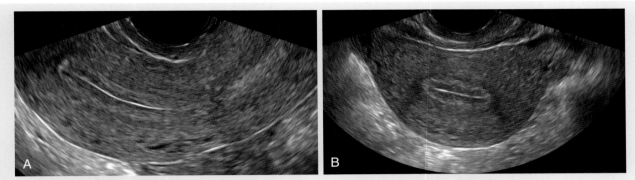

Figure II-10   A and B, The normal endometrium seen transvaginally both in longitudinal and transverse sections, showing no irregularities or focal lesions.

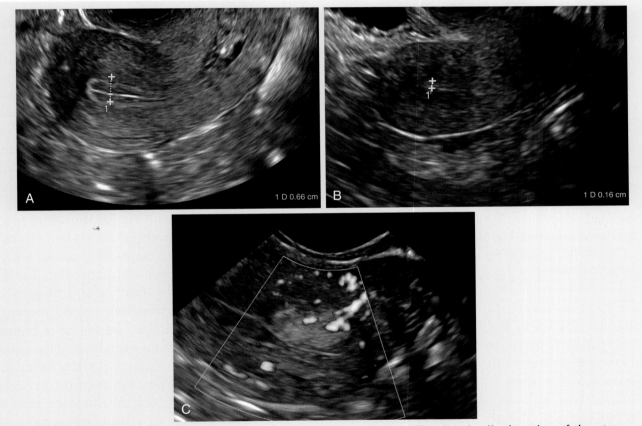

Figure II-11   ** The measurement of the endometrial echo is done in a midline longitudinal section of the uterus with the transverse axis of the uterus identical to the axis of the transducer to obtain the true sagittal view of the uterus. **A and B show the measurements done on a premenopausal and postmenopausal patient, respectively. **C** shows the presence of a focal polyp with a feeder vessel demonstrated using color Doppler. The rest of the endometrium was less than 4 mm in this postmenopausal patient with bleeding.

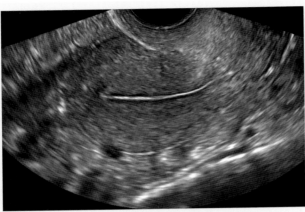

Figure II-12   Transvaginal view of a normal uterus in the early proliferative phase, showing a very thin, echogenic, and linear endometrium.

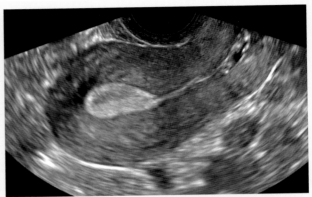

Figure II-14   Transvaginal view of the normal luteal phase endometrium, which has a homogeneous, lobular, and thickened sonographic appearance.

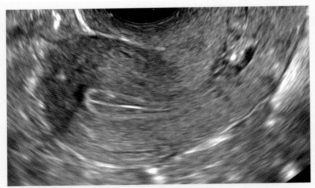

Figure II-13   Transvaginal view of the uterus in a patient who is midcycle and about to ovulate. Note the trilaminar pattern of the endometrial echo, with a thin linear echogenic line at the center surrounded by a lucent rim, which is further encircled by an echogenic basilar layer.

basilar layer (Figure II-13). The endometrium further thickens in the secretory or luteal phase and takes on a more homogeneous, lobular, and thickened appearance, which is normal before menstruation (Figure II-14).

In patients who are not cycling, the endometrium should maintain a constant appearance and is typically thin and homogeneous (Figure II-15). The measurement of the endometrial echo is not as important as the appearance and texture of the endometrium. The width can change dramatically during the cycle, and only

measurements done in the early proliferative phase are an accurate representation of the cavity. There are no true normative data of the measurement of the endometrium in premenopausal patients, and endometrial abnormalities are detected by the presence of focal abnormalities and asymmetry. Patients who have had an endometrial ablation may have a markedly heterogeneous appearance of the myometrium and endometrial-myometrial junction, making any meaningful measurement or characterization impossible. The region of the endometrium typically looks puckered and the surrounding myometrium mottled in these patients (Figure II-16).

In postmenopausal patients who are *not* bleeding, there are no accepted normative data for the width of the endometrium. The sonographic appearance of the endometrium and the presence of any abnormal color flow are far more important factors in detecting abnormalities of the endometrium. In postmenopausal patients who are bleeding, the width of the endometrium is useful in the initial evaluation. If it measures less than or equal to 4 mm and appears linear, echogenic, and straight, further testing is not typically indicated in a low-risk patient unless bleeding recurs (Figure II-17). There is disagreement as to whether the upper limit of normal should be 4 or 5 mm; however, the American College of Obstetrics and Gynecology recommends that greater than 4 mm

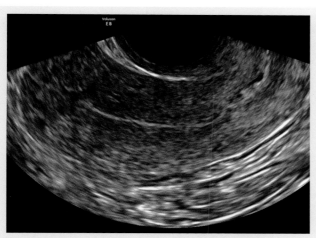

Figure II-15 Transvaginal view of the endometrium in a patient on oral contraception, showing a thin linear endometrium, which is typical of patients who are not cycling.

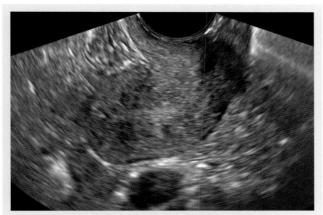

Figure II-16 Transvaginal view of the uterus of a patient who has undergone an endometrial ablation. Note the characteristic puckered look of the endometrium that is indistinct and unmeasurable. The surrounding myometrium is mottled and blotchy.

warrants further evaluation (see Endometrial Hyperplasia and the Differential Diagnosis for Thick Endometrium and also Endometrial Carcinoma). If part of the endometrium is obscured by fibroids, polyps, or adenomyosis, or if the margins are indistinct, saline infusion sonohysterography can be a useful adjunct for further evaluation (Figure II-18).

Volume imaging of the uterus (3-D) is a very helpful adjunct to 2-D ultrasound, especially when there is any perceived abnormality on standard 2-D evaluation. The coronal view of the uterus is key to detecting Müllerian duct anomalies, abnormally located IUDs, submucous fibroids, and polyps (see individual sections) (Figure II-19). If a sonohysterogram is performed, acquiring a 3-D volume during the saline infusion is invaluable for a comprehensive evaluation of the endometrial cavity offline (Figure II-20). The patency of the fallopian tubes can also be tested by injecting air mixed with saline into the uterine cavity and watching the echogenic air bubbles travel through the tubes in real-time (hysterosalpingo- contrast sonography, or HyCoSy).

The Adnexa

To evaluate the adnexa transvaginally, it is best to begin at the level of the uterine fundus in the transverse section. One can then follow the tubo-ovarian ligament out laterally toward the ovary. In most patients the ovary is located at the end of the tubo-ovarian ligament along the pelvic side wall and iliac vessels. Patients who have had pelvic surgery, endometriosis, or pelvic inflammatory disease tend to have ovaries that are in unpredictable locations and more difficult to find because of adhesions. Postmenopausal ovaries are small, lack folliculogenesis, and thus are difficult to identify in some cases (Figure II-21). In patients who had a hysterectomy, the ovaries are particularly hard to identify because of the lack of reference usually provided by the uterus. The practitioner can use his or her free hand to press on the patient's lower abdomen while scanning transvaginally much like a bimanual examination. This maneuver often shifts the abdominal organs so that the ovary can appear from behind a loop of bowel. Asking the patient to perform the Valsalva maneuver will also accomplish similar results when trying to find hidden ovaries. If the uterus is enlarged by fibroids or adenomyosis, ovaries can be undetectable sonographically. In such cases one must still evaluate the adnexa carefully to rule out masses.

The ovaries are measured in three dimensions (width, length, and depth), in two planes that

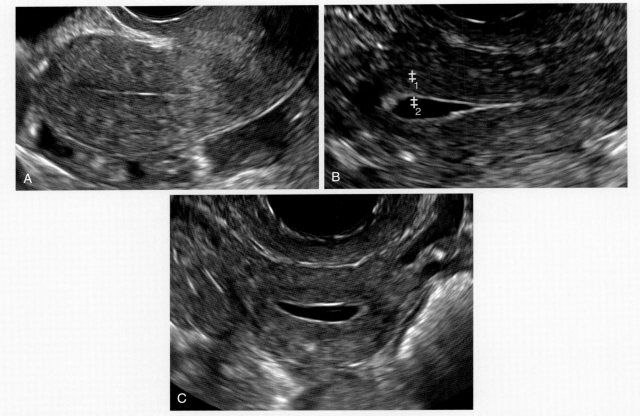

Figure II-17 **A** shows a transvaginal view of the typical paper-thin, echogenic endometrium in a postmenopausal patient. **B and C** show a small amount of fluid in the endometrial cavity of a postmenopausal patient, which is not considered clinically significant in the presence of a thin endometrium (*calipers*).

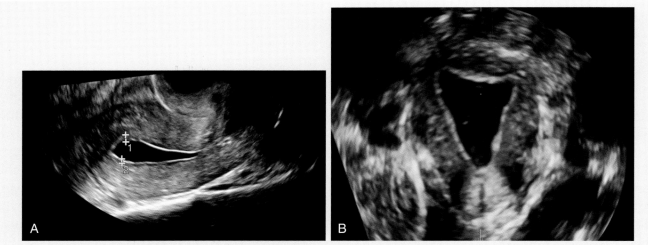

Figure II-18 **A and B,** Normal sonohysterogram seen both in 2-D and 3-D coronal reconstruction. Note the saline in the endometrial cavity outlining a thin and smooth lining.

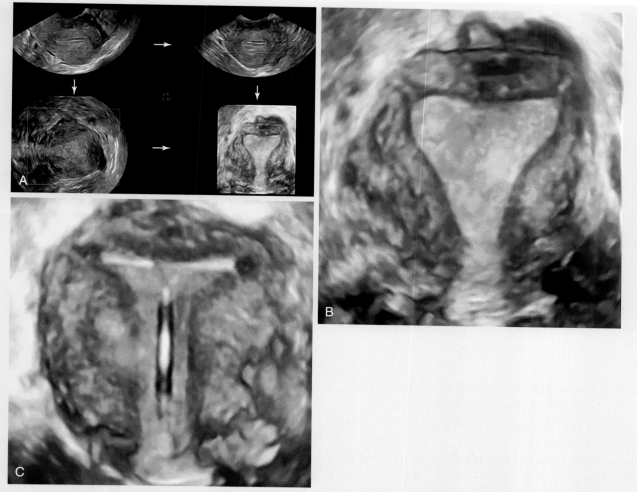

Figure II-19   3-D volume acquisitions of the uterus are essential to generate the reconstructed coronal view of the uterus. **A** shows the multiplanar display of the volume acquisition. **B** shows the reconstructed coronal view of the uterus and cavity showing a normal shape. Note that even the interstitial portions of the tubes can be visualized. **C** shows the normal positioning of an IUD within the uterine cavity.

are at right angles to each other (Figure II-22). Women who are cycling typically have one or more follicles on each ovary (up to 2.5 to 3 cm in largest diameter), particularly if examined midcycle (Figure II-23; also see the section on ovarian cysts). Postmenopausal women should not normally have ovarian cysts, although a small clear cyst less than or equal to 10 mm is considered clinically insignificant.

It is also important to evaluate the entire adnexal area, including the pelvic side wall, to identify any abnormal fluid collection or masses. The fallopian tubes are not usually seen unless abnormal or outlined by free fluid.

Color Doppler ultrasound is often helpful to determine whether an adnexal cyst or lesion is vascular. An intense circular vascular pattern indicates a corpus luteum, which is a normal finding in a cycling woman. Other masses with abundant central blood flow may be worrisome for malignancy.

The Cul-de-sac

The cul-de-sac should be evaluated for the presence of masses or free fluid behind the cervix. This is an area that is often affected by deep penetrating endometriosis in the anterior wall of the rectosigmoid (see Endometriosis). Masses in this

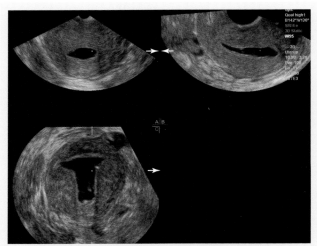

Figure II-20 Multiplanar display of the 3-D volume acquisition done during a sonohysterogram. Note that all three orthogonal views are seen simultaneously. One can navigate through the saved volume at a review station after the patient has left.

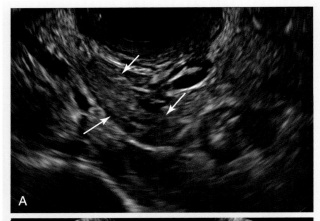

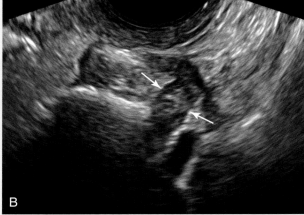

Figure II-21 **A and B,** Transvaginal view of the right and left ovary in a postmenopausal patient. Note the typical comma shape of the ovary, which is thin rather than fat and rounded, as seen premenopausally.

area may include fibroids, an enlarged ovary, a bowel lesion, or a presacral mass.

Part of the evaluation of the cul-de-sac should include testing the mobility of the uterus. The uterus can be moved slightly by gently pushing on the cervix with the vaginal probe in the vagina. If the cul-de-sac is frozen by adhesions or endometriosis, the uterus will not glide past the anterior wall of the rectosigmoid as it normally should.

Nongynecologic Organs

We must not forget that the uterus, ovaries, and fallopian tubes are not alone in the female pelvis. There are multiple loops of small and large bowel as well as the appendix, the ureters, lymph nodes, blood vessels, and sacrum. It is important to keep these organs in mind when performing pelvic ultrasound because not all masses and fluid collections are attributable to the uterus and adnexa (see related sections).

In conclusion, ultrasound is well known and accepted as the chosen method of imaging the female pelvis for practically all indications. The sonographic armamentarium at our disposal is vast and includes gray scale, 3-D volume imaging, color Doppler mapping, introduction of saline

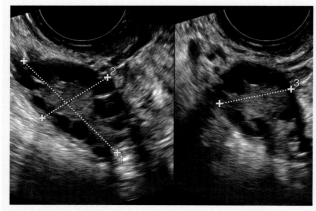

Figure II-22 Transvaginal view of a normal ovary showing the correct method of measuring the ovary.

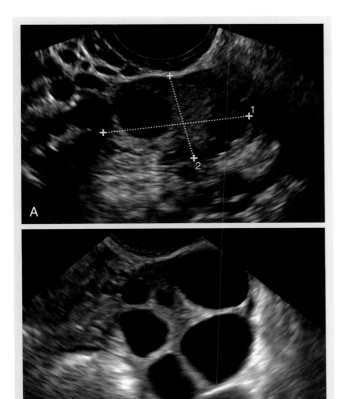

into the uterus, extended-field-of-view images, and so on. Ultrasound techniques are versatile, operator dependent, and vary with patient body habitus, previous surgery, and the anatomy of each individual patient. This differentiates sonography from other forms of cross-sectional imaging, which are standardized. Performing quality ultrasound includes deciding what images are needed, acquiring quality images, and finally interpreting them. The well-trained and experienced sonologist and/or sonographer can resolve the vast majority of gynecologic problems with ultrasound imaging.

Figure II-23 Transvaginal view of a normal ovary in two different patients. **A** shows the normal ovary as the dominant follicle is maturing mid-cycle. **B** shows multiple follicles in a patient taking Clomid for the treatment of infertility.

Section 3

Case Studies for Review

Directions: For each case study in this section, review the provided information and images and suggest a diagnosis. Actual results for each case may be found at the end of the section on pp. 264-265.

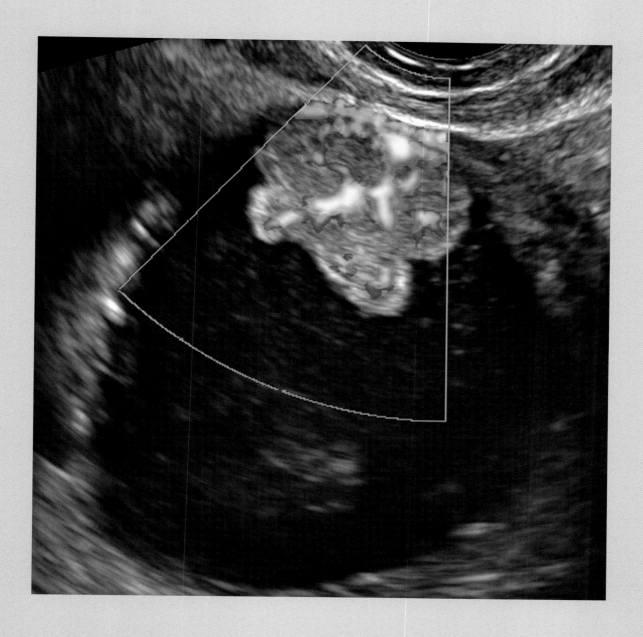

Case 1

This adnexal mass was found in a 33-year-old patient who was asymptomatic.

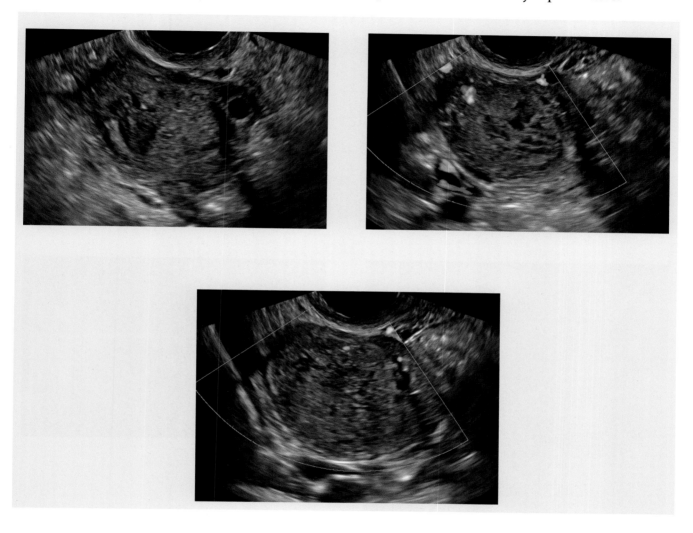

Case 2

This 48-year-old nulliparous patient had a long history of pelvic pain and dyspareunia, worse at the time of menses.

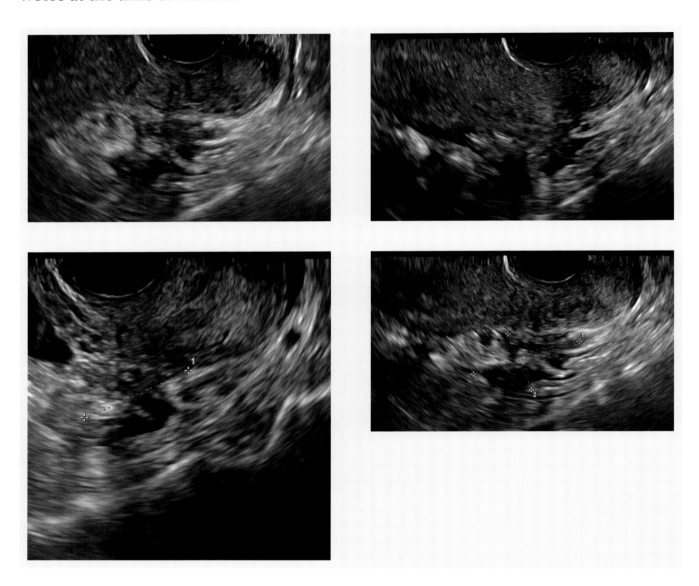

Case 3

This 57-year-old patient was referred for a second opinion of a right ovarian cyst discovered on an ultrasound at a different institution.

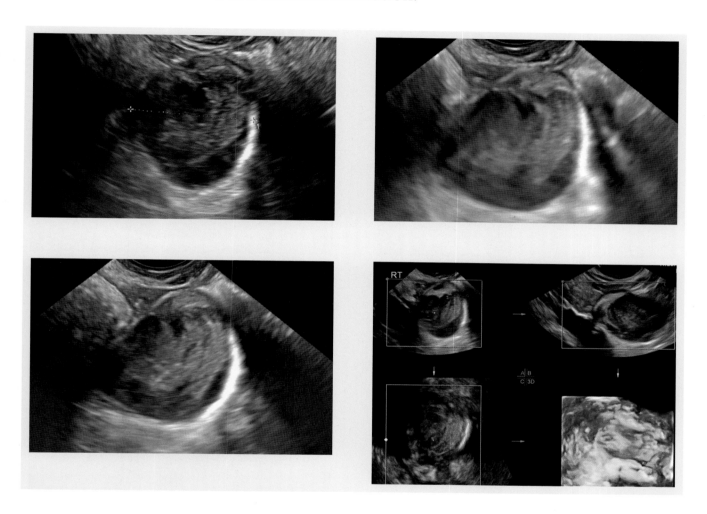

Case 4

This patient presented for a scan to evaluate the uterus due to infertility. These are images of both ovaries. The uterus was normal.

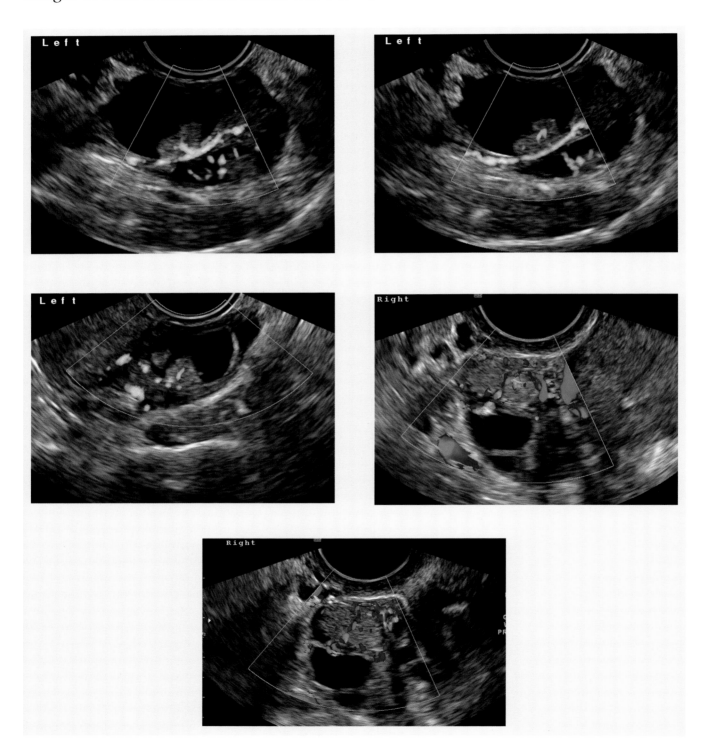

Case 5

This 66-year-old patient with breast cancer is being treated with Tamoxifen. She was referred for a sonohysterogram for evaluation of a "thickened endometrium" seen on an ultrasound done elsewhere.

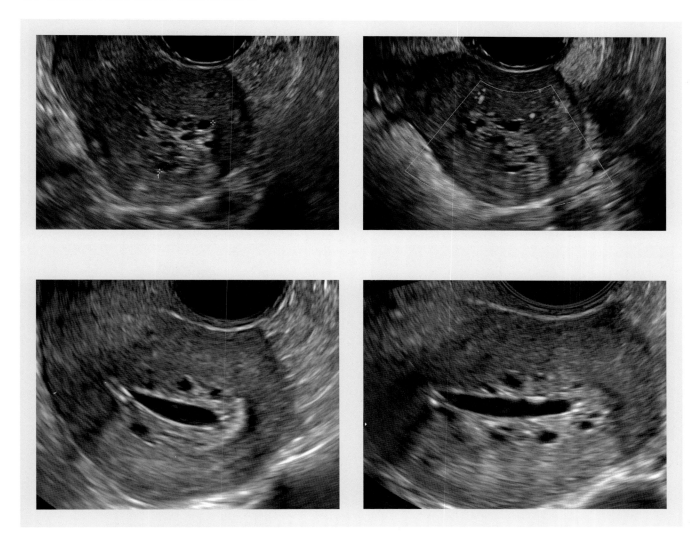

Case 6

This 72-year-old woman presented with pelvic pain on urination and urinary urgency.

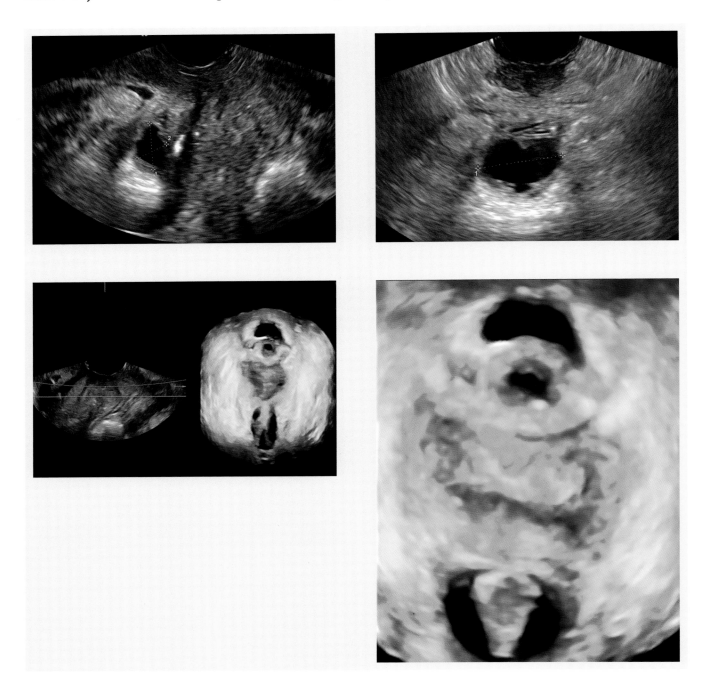

Case 7

This 36-year-old patient had a recent spontaneous abortion but has had persistent heavy bleeding for the past 3 weeks.

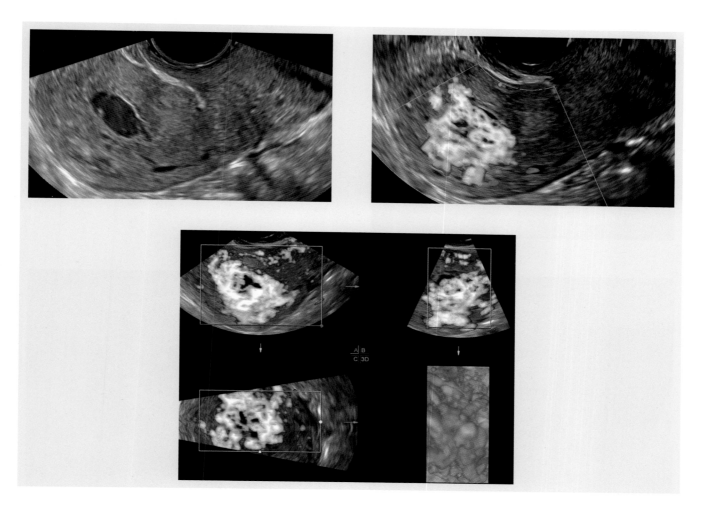

Case 8

This 32-year-old patient presented with cyclic dysuria and pelvic pain.

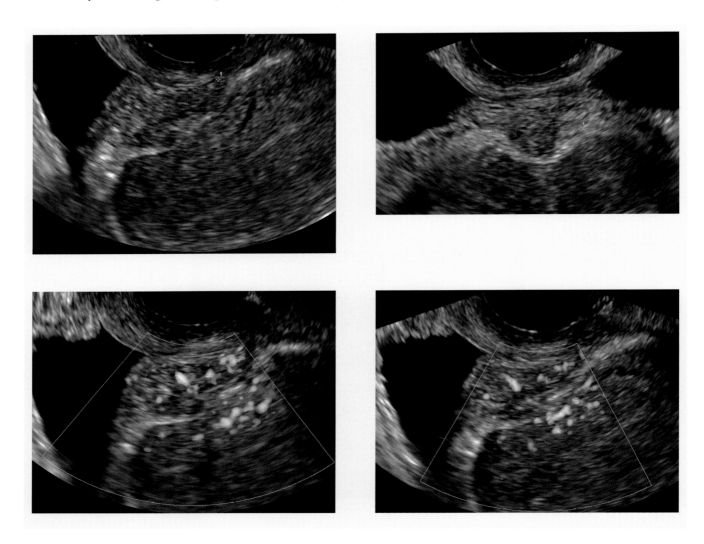

Case 9

This pelvic mass was present in the cul-de-sac of an asymptomatic 44-year-old patient. The ovaries could not be clearly identified.

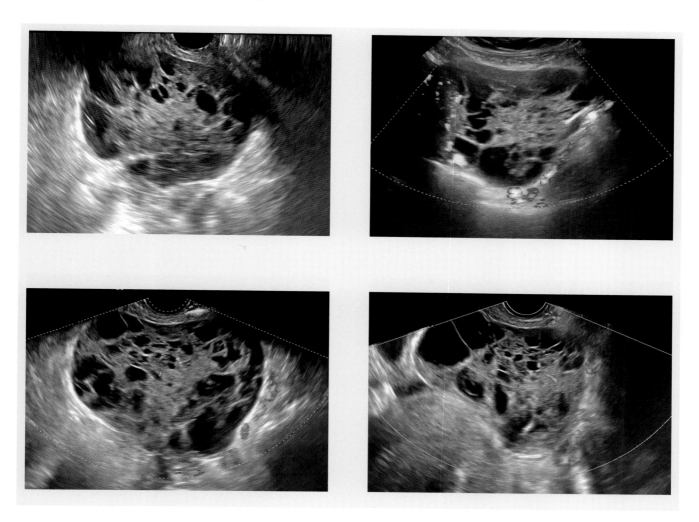

Case 10

This 69-year-old postmenopausal patient with a retroverted uterus presented with a history of recent vaginal bleeding.

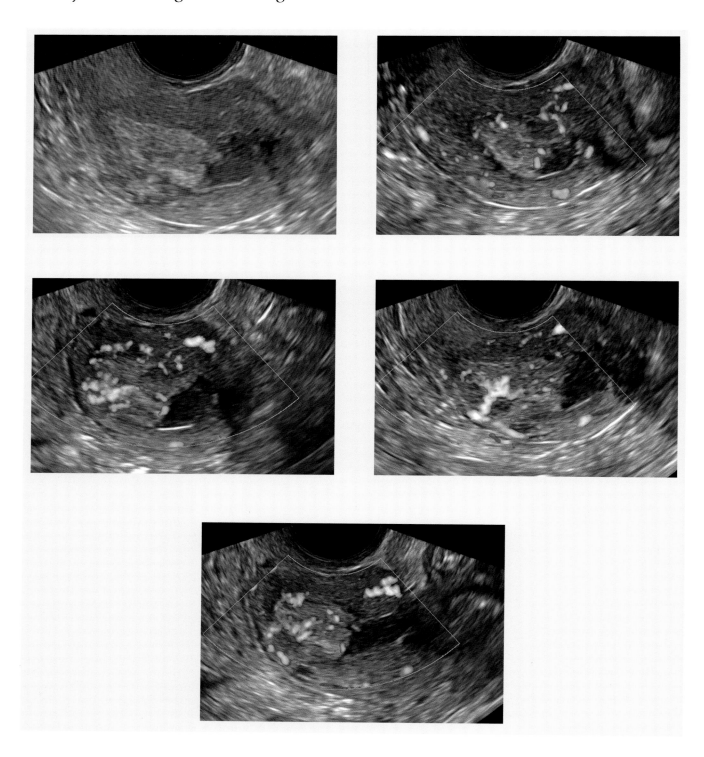

Case 11

This 27-year-old woman presented with a very large pelvic mass and ascites.

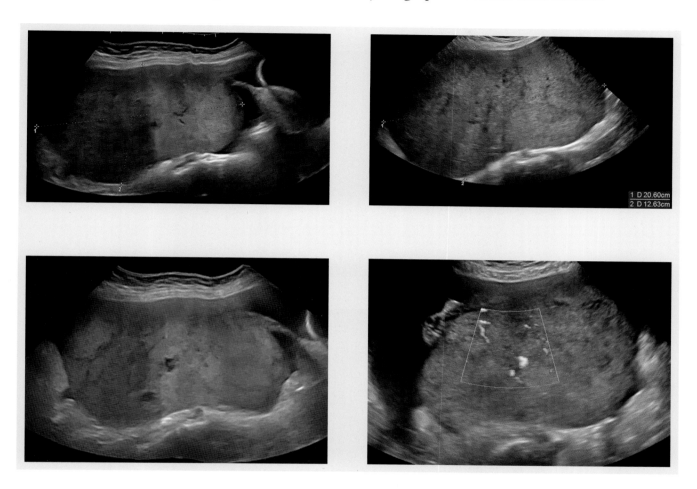

Case 12

This postmenopausal patient presented with several hours of right lower quadrant pain. The scan was done transvaginally.

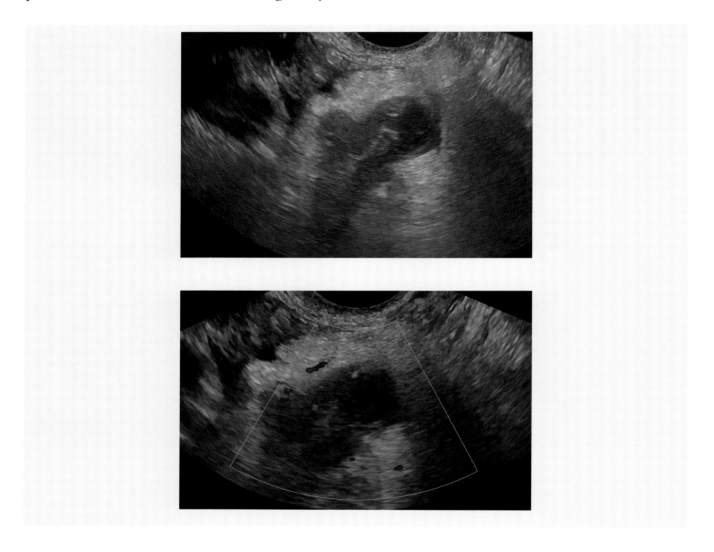

Case 13

This 56-year-old postmenopausal woman had not had a pelvic exam for decades. She was brought in by her family for a prolonged history of vaginal bleeding.

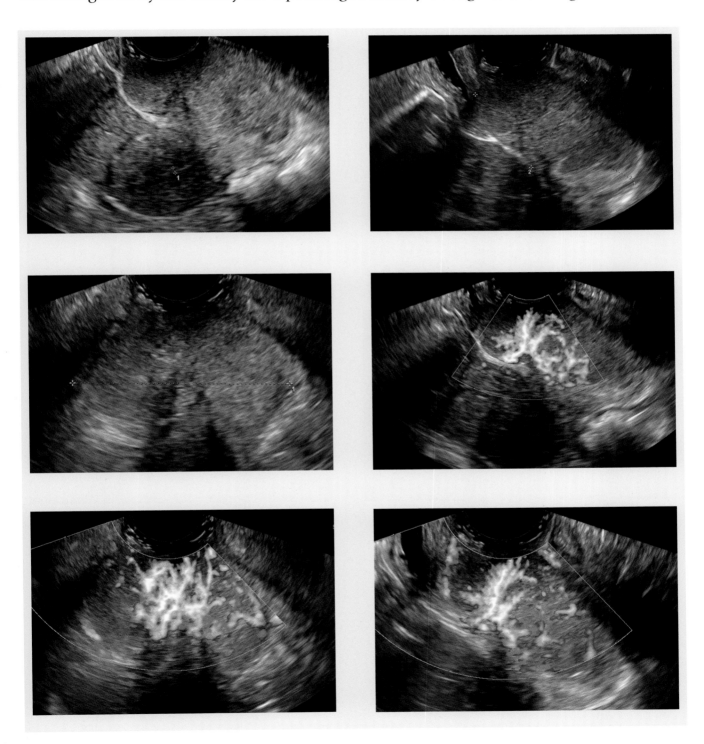

Case 14

This 37-year-old patient has a history of choriocarcinoma that was successfully treated 5 years ago. Recently, she was treated for a missed abortion with a D&C and was being seen for persistently elevated serum beta-HCG. After a second D&C procedure, the levels continued to rise and this ultrasound was done.

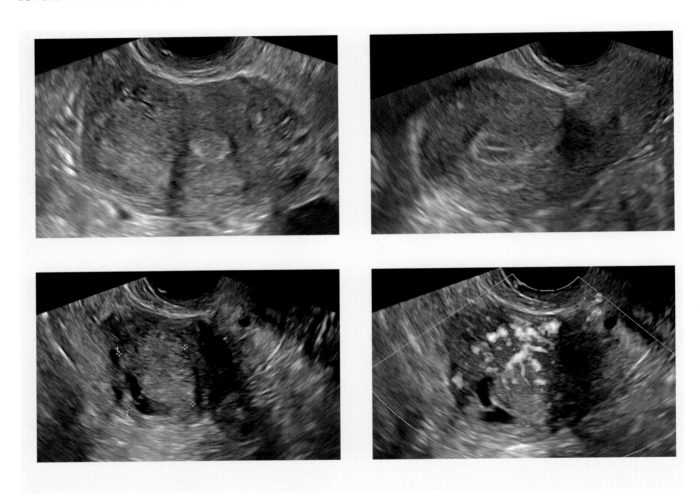

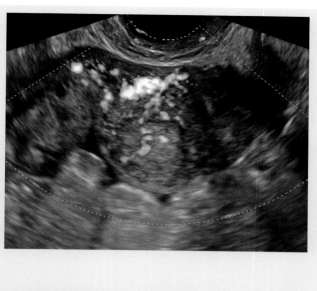

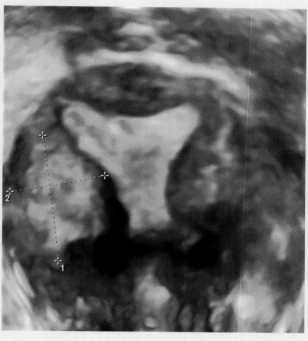

Case 15

This 28-year-old pregnant woman had a routine obstetrical ultrasound. This right ovarian mass was noted incidentally at 18 weeks.

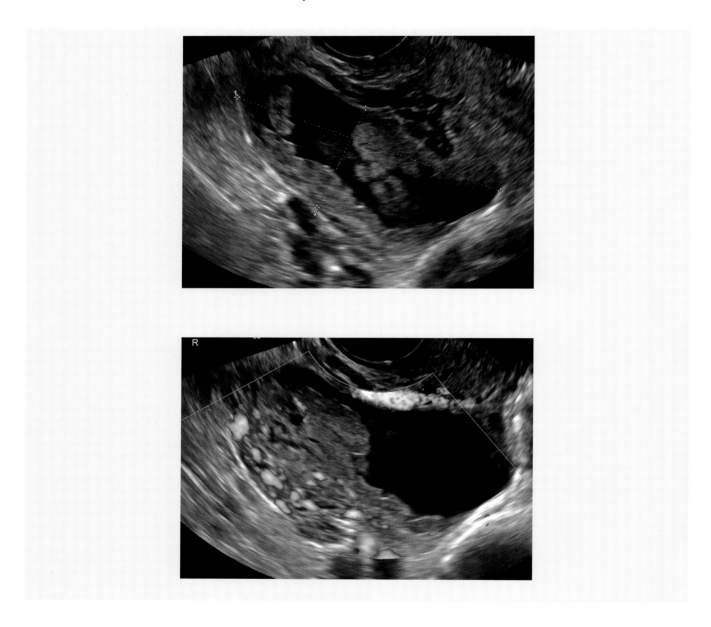

Case 16

This 36-year-old patient had a positive pregnancy test and vaginal bleeding.

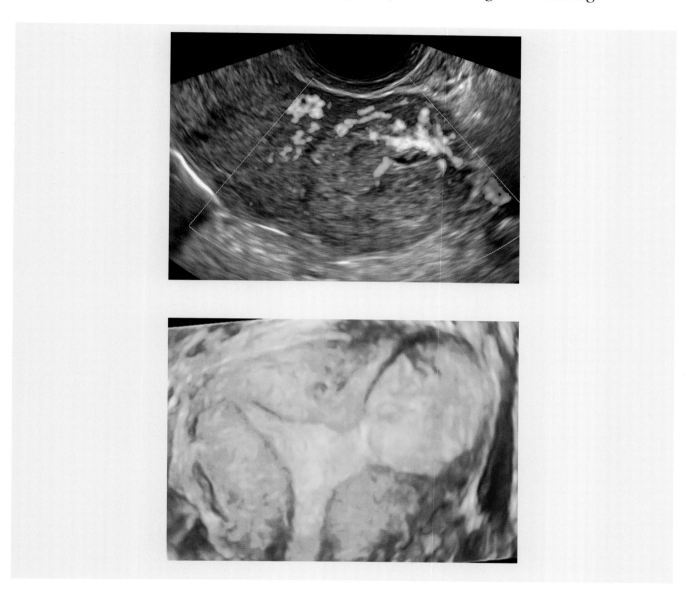

Case 17

This 66-year-old patient had dull, chronic pelvic pain. The transvaginal ultrasound shows bilateral avascular posterior pelvic masses.

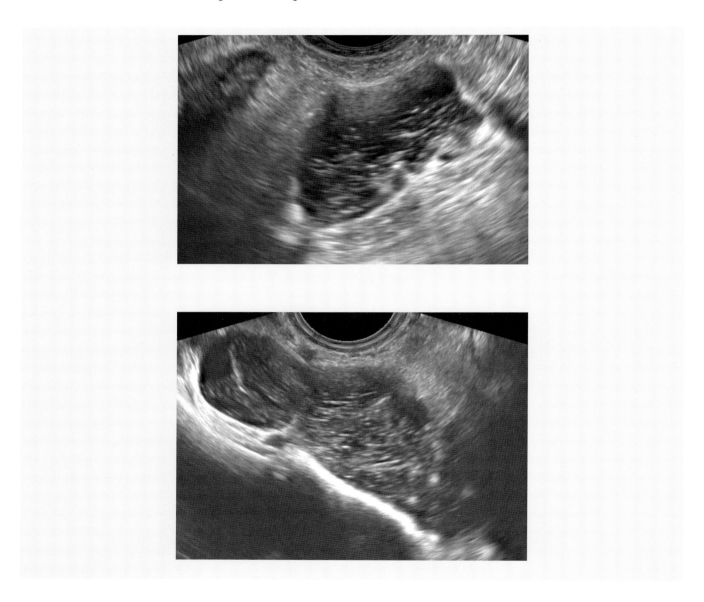

Case 18

This is an asymptomatic right adnexal mass in a 32-year-old patient. Images include both transabdominal and transvaginal views.

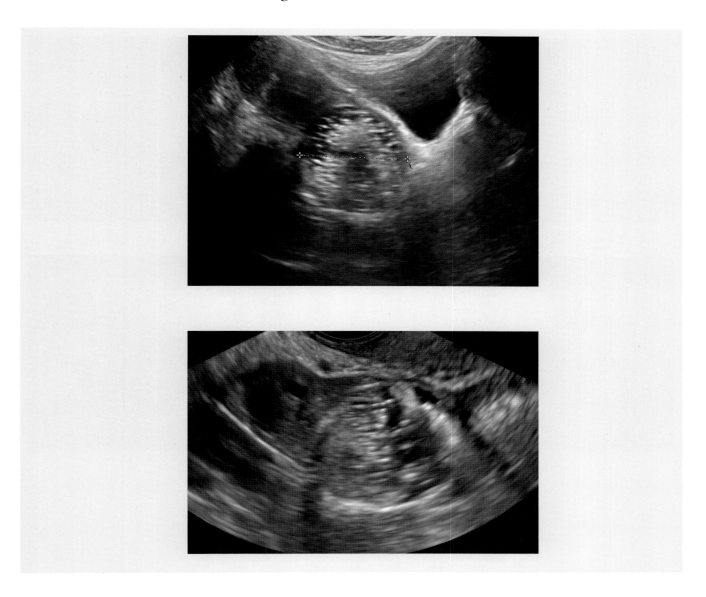

Case 19

This 44-year-old woman presented with chronic severe pelvic pain. The uterus and ovaries were normal sonographically.

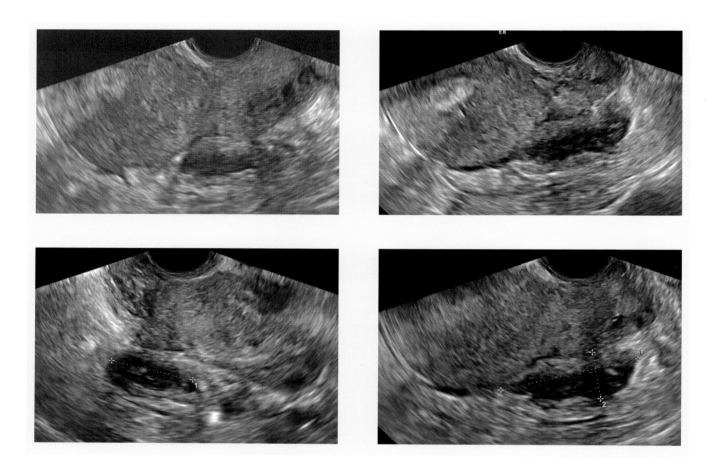

Case 20

This 37-year-old patient was referred because of a pelvic mass seen on other imaging.

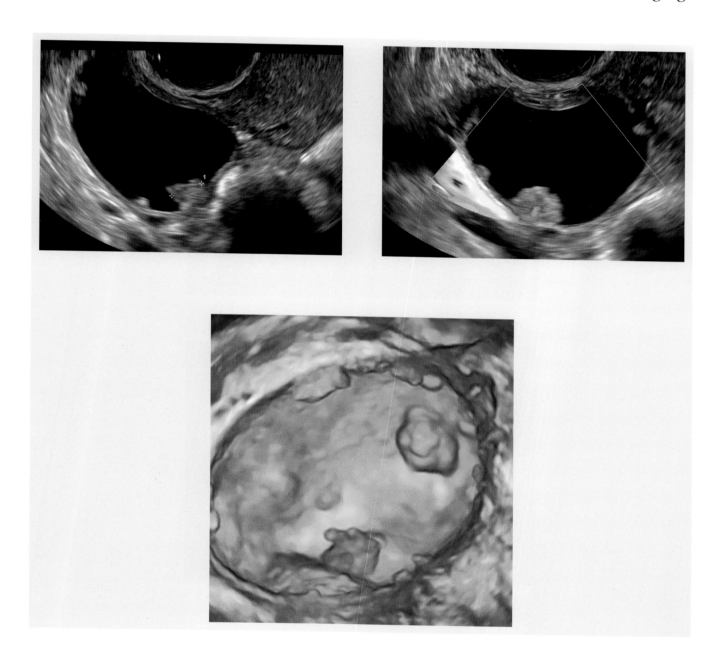

Case 21

This cystic structure was an incidental finding on a transabdominal pelvic ultrasound done on a 77-year-old woman.

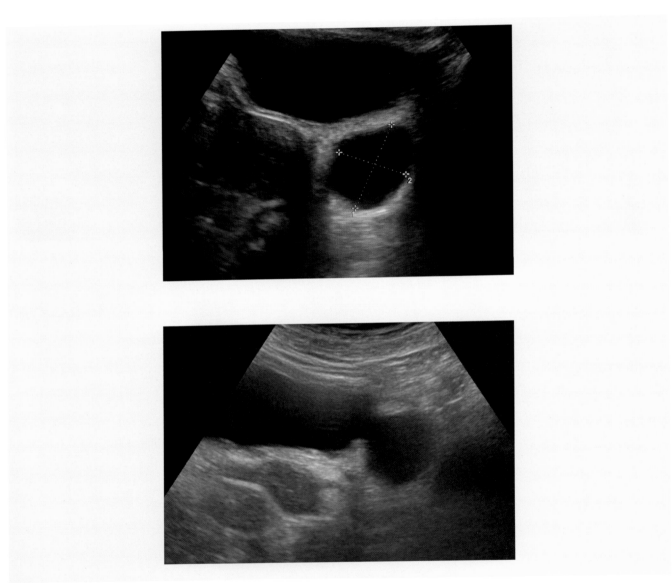

Case 22

This 48-year-old patient complained of pelvic pain, and the top two images were obtained. The patient returned 3 weeks later, and the bottom two images were obtained.

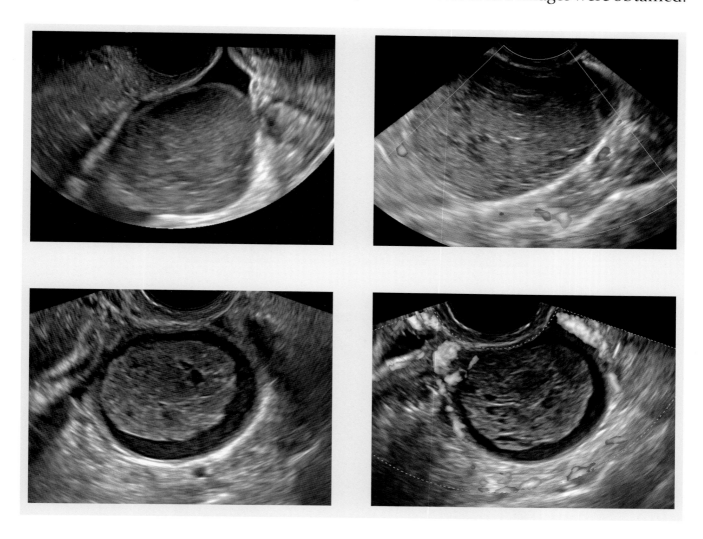

Case 23

This 64-year-old woman was sent for an ultrasound because of a family history of ovarian cancer.

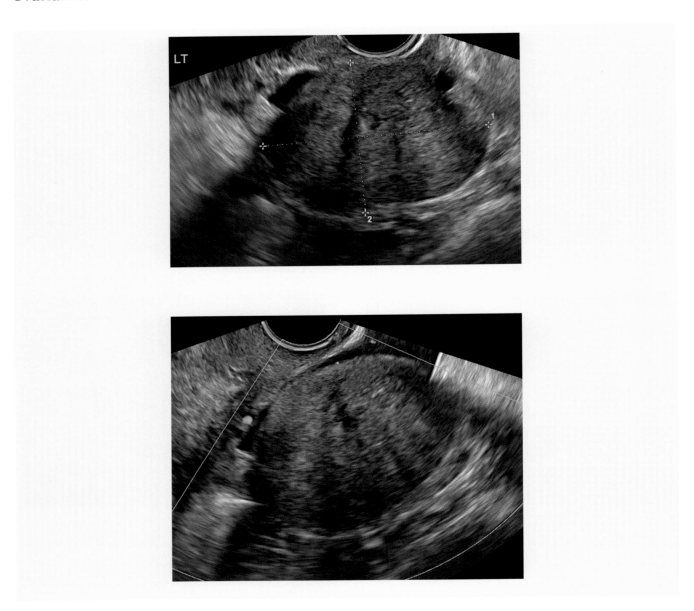

Case 24

This 33-year-old patient complained of irregular bleeding.

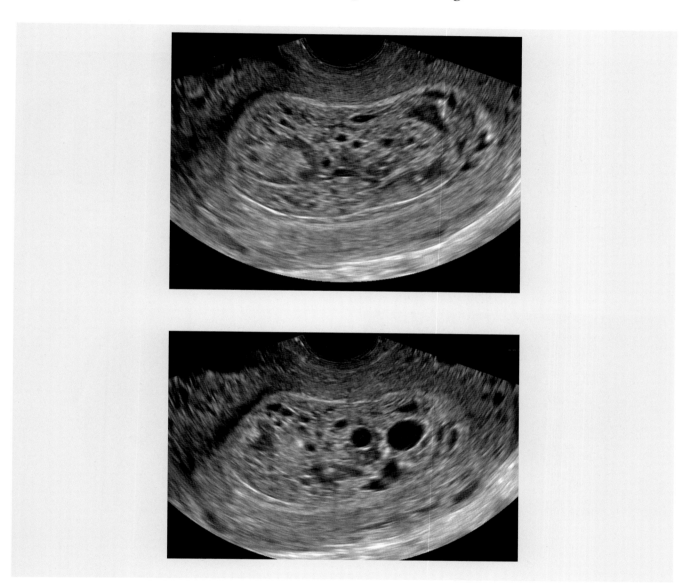

Case 25

This 51-year-old patient had a recent colonoscopy and subsequently developed pelvic pain and fever several days after the procedure.

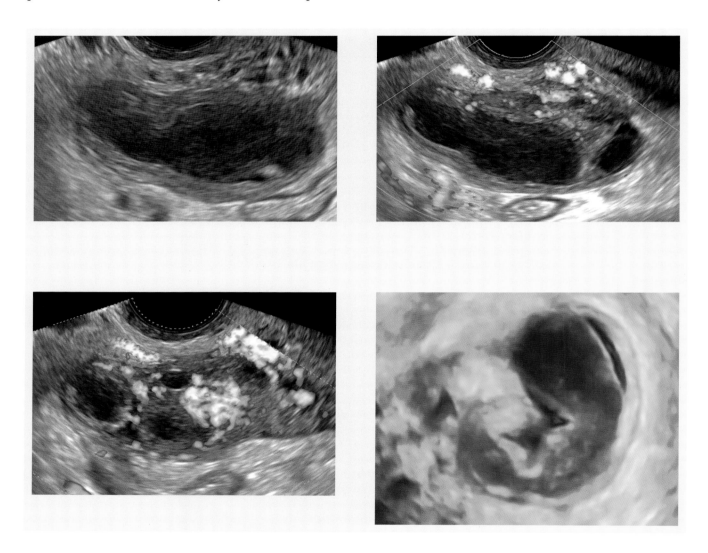

Case 26

This 25-year-old woman presented with an enlarged uterus on physical examination. The first image (top left) is a transabdominal view of the pelvis. The other images were taken transvaginally.

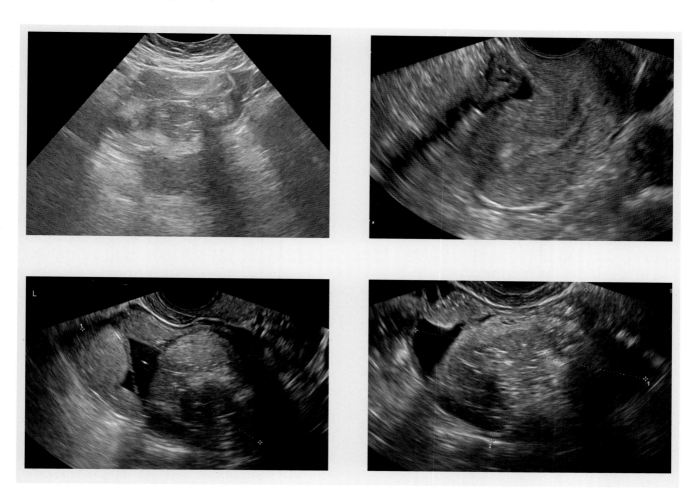

Case 1 Answer: This mass was mistaken for an ovarian fibroma but was proven to be a mature teratoma at surgery.

Case 2 Answer: Endometriosis involving the back of the cervix and anterior wall of the recto-sigmoid. There was severe focal tenderness at the site of the abnormality during the scan.

Case 3 Answer: Mucocele of the appendix. Note the onion skin–like texture of the internal contents of the lesion. A separate right ovary that appeared normal was documented.

Case 4 Answer: Bilateral cystadenomas of low malignant potential (borderline tumor). Note that these masses with abundant color flow are worrisome for malignancy.

Case 5 Answer: The initial scan suggested a polyp due to the thick, heterogeneous, and cystic central endometrial echo. When saline was infused into the uterine cavity, the mucosal surface appeared thin, compatible with atrophy. The cystic areas are sub-endometrial, which is typical of the Tamoxifen effect and represents glandular cystic atrophy.

Case 6 Answer: Urethral diverticulum. The scans were all done from the perineum, looking down the length of the urethra and vagina. The location of the diverticulum is best seen on the 3-D reconstructed view of the perineum and forms a semilunar shape around the anterior aspect of the urethra.

Case 7 Answer: Retained products of conception. Note the extreme vascularity, which is very common when the abortion is incomplete. This vascularity will resolve completely after a D&C.

Case 8 Answer: Endometriosis of the posterior bladder wall and anterior aspect of the uterus. Note the mass-like thickening of the floor of the bladder *(calipers)* with involvement of the wall of the uterus underneath.

Case 9 Answer: Degenerating fibroid. The appearance of this mass was nonspecific and more suggestive of an ovarian lesion. The correct diagnosis was not suspected preoperatively because this appearance is atypical for a fibroid, even with degeneration.

Case 10 Answer: This is a thickened endometrium, worrisome for malignancy. The final pathologic diagnosis was grade 2 endometrial adenocarcinoma. Note the vascular mass involving the endometrium and invading the anterior myometrium as well as the echogenic fluid within the cavity (blood).

Case 11 Answer: Dysgerminoma measuring 20 cm × 12 cm.

Case 12 Answer: Acute appendicitis. Note that the appendix has a cystic area in its tip and is surrounded by very echogenic tissue, which represents inflammation of the surrounding fat. A separate, normal right ovary was clearly identified.

Case 13 Answer: Large cervical carcinoma. The first image (top left) shows the measurement of the endometrium, and the second image (top right) shows the calipers on the cervical mass. Note the extreme vascularity.

Case 14 Answer: Intramural choriocarcinoma. The tumor was confined to the myometrium and not contiguous with the endometrial cavity. The patient was treated with chemotherapy to no avail and eventually underwent a hysterectomy for definitive therapy. The tissue typing of the tumor was different from the original choriocarcinoma, consistent with a second, primary choriocarcinoma as opposed to a recurrence.

Case 15 Answer: Decidualized endometrioma.

Case 16 Answer: Left cornual pregnancy. Note how the 3-D coronal image best demonstrates the location of the pregnancy.

Case 17 Answer: Tarlov's cysts along the anterior aspect of the sacrum bilaterally. The normal ovaries were identified separately.

Case 18 Answer: Right dermoid cyst.

Case 19 Answer: Nodular, deep-penetrating endometriosis of the anterior wall of the recto-sigmoid, behind the distal end of the cervix. The cul-de-sac was frozen with endometriotic implants.

Case 20 Answer: Serous cystadenoma of low malignant potential (borderline tumor). Note the few internal mural nodules containing neovascularity seen by color flow Doppler.

Case 21 Answer: Bladder diverticulum. Note the connection to the bladder on the bottom image.

Case 22 Answer: Hemorrhagic cyst with retracting clot over the course of 3 weeks. Note that the initial scan suggested a solid mass, but this was an avascular clot and was seen to retract 3 weeks later. In addition, the blood flow was only seen peripherally.

Case 23 Answer: Fibrothecoma of the ovary. Note the solid texture with limited blood flow as well as the multiple vertical shadowing stripes (Venetian blind appearance) characteristic of fibromas.

Case 24 Answer: (Hint: The patient had a positive pregnancy test). Complete molar pregnancy. Note that without the complete history, the sonographic appearance could be confused with an endometrial polyp or other endometrial process.

Case 25 Answer: Pelvic inflammatory disease with pyosalpinx. This was thought to be a complication resulting from a micro-perforation during a colonoscopy and was treated with broad-spectrum antibiotics.

Case 26 Answer: Large dermoid located above the uterine fundus. The location of the dermoid likely simulated an enlarged uterus clinically; however, the uterus was normal.

Index

A

Abdominal pregnancies, 58. *See also* Ectopic pregnancies.
Abdominal wall lesions, anterior, 77–78. *See also* Endometriosis.
Abnormal intrauterine device (IUD) locations, 109–113
  clinical aspects of, 110
  differential diagnosis for, 109
  etiology of, 109
  recommendations for, 110
  synonyms for, 109
  ultrasound findings for, 109
Abortion, incomplete, 172. *See also* Retained products of conception (RPOC).
Abscesses, tubo-ovarian (TOAs), 199–202
  clinical aspects of, 199–200
  differential diagnosis for, 199
  etiology of, 199
  vs. pelvic inflammatory disease (PID), 199–200
  recommendations for, 199–200
  synonyms for, 199
  ultrasound findings for, 199, 200f–202f
Adenocarcinomas, colon, 27. *See also* Bowel diseases.
Adenomyomas, 3. *See also* Adenomyosis.
Adenomyosis, 1–7
  adenomyomas and, 3
  clinical aspects of, 3–4
  differential diagnosis for, 3
  etiology of, 3
  generalized, 3
  recommendations for, 3–4
  synonyms for, 3
  ultrasound findings for, 3, 4f–6f
Adenosarcomas, 205. *See also* Uterine sarcomas.
Adhesions, 8–10
  clinical aspects of, 8
  differential diagnosis for, 8
  etiology of, 8
  intrauterine, 177. *See also* Asherman's syndrome.
  recommendations for, 8
  synonyms for, 8
  ultrasound findings for, 8, 9f–10f
Adnexa, intracavity scan protocols, 221, 229–231, 232f
Adnexal cysts, 155. *See also* Paratubal and para-ovarian cysts.
Adnexal torsion, 147–152
  clinical aspects of, 148
  differential diagnosis for, 147
  etiology of, 147
  recommendations for, 148
  synonyms for, 147
  ultrasound findings for, 147, 148f–151f
Agenesis, 125. *See also* Müllerian duct anomalies.
Anatomy, normal, 221–223
Anomalies, Müllerian duct, 125–135. *See also* Müllerian duct anomalies.
Anterior abdominal wall lesions, 77–78. *See also* Endometriosis.
Appendiceal mucocele, 11–13
  clinical aspects of, 11
  differential diagnosis for, 11
  etiology of, 11

Appendiceal mucocele *(Continued)*
  recommendations for, 11
  synonyms for, 11
  ultrasound findings for, 11, 12f
Appendicitis, 26. *See also* Bowel diseases.
Arcuate uterus, 125. *See also* Müllerian duct anomalies.
Asherman's syndrome, 177–181
  clinical aspects of, 178
  differential diagnosis for, 177-178
  etiology of, 177
  recommendations for, 178
  retained products of conception (RPOC) and, 177. *See also* Retained products of conception (RPOC).
  synonyms for, 177
  T-shaped uterus and, 189. *See also* T-shaped uterus.
  ultrasound findings for, 177, 178f–180f
Asymptomatic ovarian tumors, 32. *See also* Brenner tumors.
Atrophic endometrium, 14
  clinical aspects of, 14
  differential diagnosis for, 14
  etiology of, 14
  recommendations for, 14
  synonyms for, 14
  ultrasound findings for, 14, 14f
Atrophy, endometrial, 14. *See also* Atrophic endometrium.

B

Benign entities
  bladder masses, 15. *See also* Bladder masses.
  cystic mesotheliomas, 8. *See also* Adhesions.
  germ cell tumors, 56. *See also* Dermoid cysts.
  metastasizing leiomyomas, 114. *See also* Intravenous leiomyomatosis.
  ovarian tumors, 32. *See also* Brenner tumors.
Bicornuate uterus, 125. *See also* Müllerian duct anomalies.
Bladder masses, 15–20. *See also* Masses.
  clinical aspects of, 16
  differential diagnosis for, 16
  etiology of, 15
  recommendations for, 16
  synonyms for, 15
  ultrasound findings for, 15, 16f–20f
Bladder wall lesions, 77–78. *See also* Lesions.
Borderline ovarian tumor, 21–25
  clinical aspects of, 21
  differential diagnosis for, 21
  etiology of, 21
  recommendations for, 21
  synonyms for, 21
  ultrasound findings for, 21, 22f–25f
Bowel diseases, 26–31
  adenocarcinomas, colon, 27
  appendicitis, 26
  colon cancer, 27
  Crohn's disease, 26
  diverticulitis, 26–27
  duplication cysts, 27
  endometriosis, rectosigmoid colon, 26
  etiology of, 26

Bowel diseases *(Continued)*
  gastrointestinal stromal tumors (GISTs), 27
  inflammatory bowel diseases, 26
  lymphomas, 27
  synonyms for, 26
  ulcerative colitis, 26
  ultrasound findings for, 26–27, 28f–30f
BRCA 1/BRCA 2, 196
Brenner tumors, 32–33. *See also* Tumors.
  clinical aspects of, 32
  differential diagnosis for, 32
  etiology of, 32
  recommendations for, 32
  synonyms for, 32
  ultrasound findings for, 32, 32f
Bright spots, ovarian, 136. *See also* Calcifications, ovarian.

C

Calcifications, ovarian, 136
  clinical aspects of, 136
  differential diagnosis for, 136
  etiology of, 136
  recommendations for, 136
  synonyms for, 136
  ultrasound findings for, 136, 136f
Carcinomas
  adenocarcinomas, colon, 27
  endometrial, 65–70
  ovarian, 137–146. *See also* Epithelial ovarian cancer.
  primary fallopian tube (PFTCs), 196–198
  serous intraepithelial tubal carcinomas (STICs), 137
  tubal, 196
Carcinosarcomas, 205. *See also* Uterine sarcomas.
Cervical masses, 34–38. *See also* Masses.
  clinical aspects of, 35
  differential diagnosis for, 35
  etiology of, 34
  recommendations for, 35
  synonyms for, 34
  ultrasound findings for, 34, 35f–38f
Cervical pregnancies, 58. *See also* Ectopic pregnancies.
Cervix, intracavity scan protocols, 20f, 224, 225f
Cesarean section (C-section) scar defects, 39–42
  clinical aspects of, 39
  differential diagnosis for, 39
  etiology of, 39
  recommendations for, 39
  synonyms for, 39
  ultrasound findings for, 39, 40f–41f
CL. *See* Corpus luteum (CL).
Clear cysts, 48–50. *See also* Cysts.
  clinical aspects of, 48–49
  differential diagnosis for, 48
  etiology of, 48
  postmenopausal, 48
  premenopausal, 48
  recommendations for, 48–49
  synonyms for, 48
  ultrasound findings for, 48, 49f–50f
Colitis, ulcerative, 26. *See also* Bowel diseases.

Page numbers followed by *f* indicate figures.

Colon adenocarcinomas, 27. *See also* Bowel
   diseases.
Colon cancer, 27. *See also* Bowel diseases.
Conditions
   abscesses, tubo-ovarian (TOAs), 199–202
   adenomyosis, 1–7
   adhesions, 8–10
   bowel diseases, 26–31
   calcifications, ovarian, 136
   carcinomas
      endometrial, 65–70
      primary fallopian tube (PFTCs), 196–198
   Cesarean section (C-section) scar defects,
      39–42
   corpus luteum (CL), 43–47
   cystadenofibromas, 51–52
   cystadenomas
      mucinous, 122–124
      serous, 184–185
   cysts
      clear, 48–50
      dermoid, 53–55
      epidermoid, 83–84
      paraovarian, 155–156
      paratubal, 155–156
      peritoneal inclusion, 8–10
      Tarlov, 192–193
      theca lutein, 194–195
   dehiscence, uterine, 39–42
   dysgerminomas, 56–57
   edema, massive, 147–152
   endometriosis, 76–82
   endometrium, atrophic, 14
   fibroids, 85–92
   fibromas
      cystadenofibromas, 51–52
      ovarian, 93–95
   fibrothecomas, 93–95
   hematocolpos, 98–103
   hematometra, 98–103
   hematuria, 15–20
   hydrosalpinx, 104–108
   hyperplasia, endometrial, 71–75
   intrauterine device (IUD) locations, abnormal,
      109–113
   leiomyomatosis, intravenous, 114–115
   lymph nodes, enlarged, 116–117
   masses
      bladder, 15–20
      cervical, 34–38
      vaginal, 209–218
   mucocele, appendiceal, 11–13
   Müllerian duct abnormalities, 125–135
   ovarian cancer
      borderline, 21–25
      epithelial, 137–146
   pelvic inflammatory disease (PID), 199–202
   pelvic kidney, 159–160
   polycystic ovaries, 161–162
   polyps, endometrial, 163–169
   pregnancies, ectopic, 58–64
   premature ovarian failure, 170–171
   retained products of conception (RPOC),
      172–176
   sarcomas, uterine, 205–208
   Schwannomas, 182–183
   stones, ureteral, 203–204
   struma ovarii, 186–188
   syndromes
      Asherman's, 177–181
      pelvic congestion, 157–158
   thecomas, 93–95
   thick endometrium, differential diagnosis,
      71–75
   torsion
      ovarian, 147–152
      tubal, 147–152

Conditions *(Continued)*
   tumors
      Brenner, 32–33
      granulosa cell (GCTs), 96–97
      metastatic to ovaries, 118–121
      uterus, T-shaped, 189–191
      vein thrombosis, ovarian, 153–154
Congenital uterine anomalies, 125. *See also*
   Müllerian duct anomalies.
Cornual pregnancies, 58. *See also* Ectopic
   pregnancies.
Corpus luteum (CL), 43–47
   clinical aspects of, 44
   differential diagnosis for, 43–44
   etiology of, 43
   recommendations for, 44
   synonyms for, 43
   ultrasound findings for, 43, 44f–47f
Crohn's disease, 26. *See also* Bowel diseases.
C-section scar defects. *See* Cesarean section
   (C-section) scar defects.
Cul-de-sac, intracavity scan protocols, 225f,
   231–232
Cystadenofibromas, 51–52
   clinical aspects of, 51
   differential diagnosis for, 51
   etiology of, 51
   recommendations for, 51
   synonyms for, 51
   ultrasound findings for, 51, 51f–52f
Cystadenomas
   mucinous, 122–124
      clinical aspects of, 122–123
      differential diagnosis for, 122
      etiology of, 122
      recommendations for, 122–123
      synonyms for, 122
      ultrasound findings for, 122, 123f
   serous, 184–185
      clinical aspects of, 184
      differential diagnosis for, 184
      etiology of, 184
      recommendations for, 184
      synonyms for, 184
      ultrasound findings for, 184, 184f–185f
Cystic mesotheliomas, benign, 8. *See also*
   Adhesions.
Cystic teratomas, mature, 53. *See also* Dermoid cysts.
Cysts
   clear, 48–50
   dermoid, 53–55
   duplication, 27
   epidermoid, 83–84
   nonfunctional, 43
   paraovarian, 155–156
   paratubal, 155–156
   peritoneal inclusion, 8–10
   Tarlov, 192–193
   theca lutein, 194–195
   vaginal, 209

D
Decidualized endometriomas, 76–77. *See also*
   Endometriosis.
Deep penetrating bowel wall/pelvic implants,
   77–78. *See also* Endometriosis.
Degenerating fibroids, 85. *See also* Fibroids.
Dehiscence, uterine, 39–42
   clinical aspects of, 39
   differential diagnosis for, 39
   etiology of, 39
   recommendations for, 39
   synonyms for, 39
   ultrasound findings for, 39, 40f–41f
Dermoid cysts, 53–55. *See also* Cysts.
   clinical aspects of, 53–54
   differential diagnosis for, 53

Dermoid cysts *(Continued)*
   etiology of, 53
   recommendations for, 53–54
   synonyms for, 53
   ultrasound findings for, 53, 54f–55f
DES. *See* Diethylstilbestrol (DES).
Didelphic uterus, 125. *See also* Müllerian duct
   anomalies.
Diethylstilbestrol (DES), 189
Diffuse bladder wall thickening. *See* Bladder
   masses
Disinfection, probes, 221–222
Distended fluid-filled fallopian tubes, 104. *See also*
   Hydrosalpinx.
Diverticula, urethral, 15. *See also* Bladder masses.
Diverticulitis, 26–27. *See also* Bowel diseases.
Duplication cysts, 27. *See also* Bowel diseases.
Dysgerminomas, 56–57
   clinical aspects of, 56
   differential diagnosis for, 56
   etiology of, 56
   recommendations for, 56
   synonyms for, 56
   ultrasound findings for, 56, 57f

E
Early menopause, 170. *See also* Premature ovarian
   failure (POF).
Ectopic kidney, 159. *See also* Pelvic kidney.
Ectopic pregnancies, 58–64
   clinical aspects of, 59
   differential diagnosis for, 59
   etiology of, 58
   recommendations for, 59
   synonyms for, 58
   ultrasound findings for, 58–59, 60f–64f
Edema, massive, 147–152
   clinical aspects of, 148
   differential diagnosis for, 147
   etiology of, 147
   recommendations for, 148
   synonyms for, 147
   ultrasound findings for, 147, 148f–151f
Endometrial atrophy, 14. *See also* Atrophic
   endometrium.
Endometrial carcinomas, 65–70. *See also*
   Carcinomas.
   clinical aspects of, 66
   differential diagnosis for, 65–66
   etiology of, 65
   recommendations for, 66
   synonyms for, 65
   ultrasound findings for, 65, 66f–70f
Endometrial hyperplasia, 71–75
   clinical aspects of, 72–75
   differential diagnosis for, 71–72
   etiology of, 71
   recommendations for, 72–75
   synonyms for, 71
Endometrial polyps, 163–169
   clinical aspects of, 163
   differential diagnosis for, 163
   etiology of, 163
   recommendations for, 163
   synonyms for, 163
   ultrasound findings for, 163, 164f–169f
Endometrial proliferation, 71. *See also* Endometrial
   hyperplasia.
Endometrial stromal tumors, 205. *See also* Uterine
   sarcomas.
Endometriomas, 76–77. *See also* Endometriosis.
Endometriosis, 76–82
   bladder masses and, 15. *See also* Bladder masses.
   clinical aspects of, 78
   differential diagnosis for, 77–78
   etiology of, 76
   of myometrium, 3. *See also* Adenomyosis.

Endometriosis (*Continued*)
  recommendations for, 78
  of rectosigmoid colon, 26. *See also* Bowel
      diseases.
  synonyms for, 76
  ultrasound findings for, 76–77, 78f–82f
  of uterus, 3. *See also* Adenomyosis.
Endometrium
  anatomy, normal, 221–223
  atrophic, 14
    clinical aspects of, 14
    differential diagnosis for, 14
    etiology of, 14
    recommendations for, 14
    synonyms for, 14
    ultrasound findings for, 14, 14f
  intracavity scan protocols, 224–229, 227f–228f
  thick, differential diagnosis, 71–75
Enlarged lymph nodes, 116–117
  clinical aspects of, 116
  differential diagnosis for, 116
  etiology of, 116
  recommendations for, 116
  synonyms for, 116
  ultrasound findings for, 116, 116f–117f
Entities
  abscesses, tubo-ovarian (TOAs), 199–202
  adenomyosis, 1–7
  adhesions, 8–10
  bowel diseases, 26–31
  calcifications, ovarian, 136
  carcinomas
    endometrial, 65–70
    primary fallopian tube (PFTCs), 196–198
  Cesarean section (C-section) scar defects, 39–42
  corpus luteum (CL), 43–47
  cystadenofibromas, 51–52
  cystadenomas
    mucinous, 122–124
    serous, 184–185
  cysts
    clear, 48–50
    dermoid, 53–55
    epidermoid, 83–84
    paraovarian, 155–156
    paratubal, 155–156
    peritoneal inclusion, 8–10
    Tarlov, 192–193
    theca lutein, 194–195
  dehiscence, uterine, 39–42
  dysgerminomas, 56–57
  edema, massive, 147–152
  endometriosis, 76–82
  endometrium, atrophic, 14
  fibroids, 85–92
  fibromas
    cystadenofibromas, 51–52
    ovarian, 93–95
  fibrothecomas, 93–95
  hematocolpos, 98–103
  hematometra, 98–103
  hematuria, 15–20
  hydrosalpinx, 104–108
  hyperplasia, endometrial, 71–75
  intrauterine device (IUD) locations, abnormal,
      109–113
  leiomyomatosis, intravenous, 114–115
  lymph nodes, enlarged, 116–117
  masses
    bladder, 15–20
    cervical, 34–38
    vaginal, 209–218
  mucocele, appendiceal, 11–13
  Müllerian duct abnormalities, 125–135
  ovarian cancer
    borderline, 21–25
    epithelial, 137–146

Entities (*Continued*)
  pelvic inflammatory disease (PID), 199–202
  pelvic kidney, 159–160
  polycystic ovaries, 161–162
  polyps, endometrial, 163–169
  pregnancies, ectopic, 58–64
  premature ovarian failure, 170–171
  retained products of conception (RPOC),
      172–176
  sarcomas, uterine, 205–208
  Schwannomas, 182–183
  stones, ureteral, 203–204
  struma ovarii, 186–188
  syndromes
    Asherman's, 177–181
    pelvic congestion, 157–158
  thecomas, 93–95
  thick endometrium, differential diagnosis,
      71–75
  torsion
    ovarian, 147–152
    tubal, 147–152
  tumors
    Brenner, 32–33
    granulosa cell (GCTs), 96–97
    metastatic to ovaries, 118–121
  uterus, T-shaped, 189–191
  vein thrombosis, ovarian, 153–154
Epidermoid cysts, 83–84. *See also* Cysts.
  clinical aspects of, 83
  differential diagnosis for, 83
  etiology of, 83
  recommendations for, 83
  synonyms for, 83
  ultrasound findings for, 83, 83f–84f
Epithelial ovarian cancer, 137–146. *See also* Ovar-
    ian cancer.
  clinical aspects of, 138
  differential diagnosis for, 138
  etiology of, 137
  recommendations for, 138
  synonyms for, 137
  ultrasound findings for, 11, 137–138,
      139f–145f
Epithelial-stromal cystic tumors, 184. *See also*
    Serous cystadenomas.

F
Fallopian tubes
  anatomy, normal, 221–223
  fluid-filled distended, 104. *See also*
      Hydrosalpinx.
  intracavity scan protocols, 223–232. *See also*
      Intracavity scan protocols.
Fibroids, 85–92
  clinical aspects of, 86
  degenerating, 85
  differential diagnosis for, 86
  etiology of, 85
  intramural, 85
  pedunculated, 85
  recommendations for, 86
  submucous, 85
  subserosal, 85
  synonyms for, 85
  ultrasound findings for, 56, 85, 91f
Fibromas
  bladder, 15. *See also* Bladder masses.
  cystadenofibromas, 51–52
    clinical aspects of, 51
    differential diagnosis for, 51
    etiology of, 51
    recommendations for, 51
    synonyms for, 51
    ultrasound findings for, 51, 51f–52f
  ovarian
    clinical aspects of, 93

Fibromas (*Continued*)
    cystadenofibromas, 51–52
    differential diagnosis for, 93
    etiology of, 93
    ovarian, 93–95
    recommendations for, 93
    synonyms for, 93
    ultrasound findings for, 93, 93f–95f
Fibromyomas, 85. *See also* Fibroids.
Fibrothecomas, 93–95
  clinical aspects of, 93
  differential diagnosis for, 93
  etiology of, 93
  recommendations for, 93
  synonyms for, 93
  ultrasound findings for, 93, 93f–95f
Fluid-filled distended fallopian tubes, 104. *See also*
    Hydrosalpinx.
Focal bladder lesions, 15. *See also* Bladder masses.

G
Gastrointestinal stromal tumors (GISTs), 27. *See
    also* Bowel diseases.
GCTs. *See* Granulosa cell tumors (GCTs).
Generalized adenomyosis, 3. *See also*
    Adenomyosis.
Germ cell tumors. *See also* Tumors.
  benign, 56. *See also* Dermoid cysts.
  malignant, 56. *See also* Dysgerminomas.
GISTs. *See* Gastrointestinal stromal tumors (GISTs).
Granulosa cell tumors (GCTs), 96–97. *See also*
    Tumors.
  clinical aspects of, 96
  differential diagnosis for, 96
  etiology of, 96
  recommendations for, 96
  synonyms for, 96
  ultrasound findings for, 96, 97f
Granulosa-theca cell tumors, 96. *See also* Granu-
    losa cell tumors (GCTs).
Gynecologic ultrasound
  of entities
    abscesses, tubo-ovarian (TOAs), 199–202
    adenomyosis, 1–7
    adhesions, 8–10
    bowel diseases, 26–31
    calcifications, ovarian, 136
    carcinomas, endometrial, 65–70
    carcinomas, primary fallopian tube (PFTCs),
        196–198
    Cesarean section (C-section) scar defects,
        39–42
    corpus luteum (CL), 43–47
    cystadenofibromas, 51–52
    cystadenomas, mucinous, 122–124
    cystadenomas, serous, 184–185
    cysts, clear, 48–50
    cysts, dermoid, 53–55
    cysts, epidermoid, 83–84
    cysts, paraovarian, 155–156
    cysts, paratubal, 155–156
    cysts, peritoneal inclusion, 8–10
    cysts, Tarlov, 192–193
    cysts, theca lutein, 194–195
    dehiscence, uterine, 39–42
    dysgerminomas, 56–57
    edema, massive, 147–152
    endometriosis, 76–82
    endometrium, atrophic, 14
    endometrium, thick (differential diagnosis),
        71–75
    fibroids, 85–92
    fibromas, ovarian, 93–95
    fibrothecomas, 93–95
    hematocolpos, 98–103
    hematometra, 98–103
    hematuria, 15–20

Gynecologic ultrasound (Continued)
    hydrosalpinx, 104–108
    hyperplasia, endometrial, 71–75
    intrauterine device (IUD) locations, abnormal, 109–113
    leiomyomatosis, intravenous, 114–115
    lymph nodes, enlarged, 116–117
    masses, bladder, 15–20
    masses, cervical, 34–38
    masses, vaginal, 209–218
    mucocele, appendiceal, 11–13
    Müllerian duct abnormalities, 125–135
    ovarian cancer, epithelial, 137–146
    ovarian tumor, borderline, 21–25
    pelvic inflammatory disease (PID), 199–202
    pelvic kidney, 159–160
    polycystic ovaries, 161–162
    polyps, endometrial, 163–169
    pregnancies, ectopic, 58–64
    premature ovarian failure, 170–171
    retained products of conception (RPOC), 172–176
    sarcomas, uterine, 205–208
    Schwannomas, 182–183
    stones, ureteral, 203–204
    struma ovarii, 186–188
    syndrome, Asherman's, 177–181
    syndrome, pelvic congestion, 157–158
    thecomas, 93–95
    torsion, ovarian, 147–152
    torsion, tubal, 147–152
    tumors, Brenner, 32–33
    tumors, granulosa cell (GCTs), 96–97
    tumors, metastatic to ovaries, 118–121
    uterus, T-shaped, 189–191
    vein thrombosis, ovarian, 153–154
    normal pelvic scans and variants, 219–234
        anatomy, normal, 221–223
        intracavity scan protocols, 223–232. See also Intracavity scan protocols.
        nongynecologic organs, 232–233
        quality-related considerations of, 232–233
        techniques, 221–223. See also Techniques.

H
hCG. See Human chorionic gonadotropin (hCG).
Hematocolpos. See Hematometra and hematocolpos.
Hematometra and hematocolpos, 98–103
    clinical aspects of, 99
    differential diagnosis for, 99
    etiology of, 98
    recommendations for, 99
    synonyms for, 98
    ultrasound findings for, 97f, 98–99, 100f–102f
Hematuria, 15–20
    clinical aspects of, 16
    differential diagnosis for, 16
    etiology of, 15
    recommendations for, 16
    synonyms for, 15
    ultrasound findings for, 15, 16f–20f
Human chorionic gonadotropin (hCG), 194
Hydrocolpos, 98. See also Hematometra and hematocolpos.
Hydrometra, 98. See also Hematometra and hematocolpos.
Hydrosalpinx, 104–108
    clinical aspects of, 105
    differential diagnosis for, 104–105
    etiology of, 104
    recommendations for, 105
    synonyms for, 104
    ultrasound findings for, 104, 105f–108f
Hyperplasia, endometrial
    clinical aspects of, 72–75

Hyperplasia, endometrial (Continued)
    differential diagnosis for, 71–72
    etiology of, 71
    recommendations for, 72–75
    synonyms for, 71
    ultrasound findings for, 71, 73f–75f
Hyperplastic polyps, 163
Hyperreactio luteinalis, 194. See also Theca lutein cysts.

I
Implants, deep penetrating bowel wall/pelvic, 77–78. See also Endometriosis.
Inclusion cysts, peritoneal, 8–10. See also Cysts.
Incomplete abortion, 172. See also Retained products of conception (RPOC).
Infections, pelvic, 199. See also Pelvic inflammatory disease (PID).
Inflammatory bowel diseases, 26. See also Bowel diseases.
Insufficiency, ovarian, 170. See also Premature ovarian failure (POF).
International Ovarian Tumor Analysis (IOTA) multicenter group, 138
Intracavity scan protocols, 221–223
    adnexa, 221, 229–231, 232f
    cervix, 20f, 224, 225f
    cul-de-sac, 225f, 231–232
    endometrium, 224–229, 227f–228f
    myometrium, 225–226
    techniques for, 221–223
        probe disinfection, 221–222
        transabdominal (TA) scans, 221–223, 222f
        transrectal (TR) scans, 222, 223f
        transvaginal (TV) scans, 221–223, 223f
    uterus, 221, 222f–223f, 224–229, 225f–226f
    vagina, 223–224, 224f
Intramural fibroids, 85. See also Fibroids.
Intrauterine adhesions, 177. See also Asherman's syndrome.
Intrauterine device (IUD) locations, abnormal, 109–113
    clinical aspects of, 110
    differential diagnosis for, 109
    etiology of, 109
    recommendations for, 110
    synonyms for, 109
    ultrasound findings for, 109
Intravenous leiomyomatosis, 114–115
    clinical aspects of, 115
    differential diagnosis for, 115
    etiology of, 114
    recommendations for, 115
    synonyms for, 114
    ultrasound findings for, 114
IOTA. See International Ovarian Tumor Analysis (IOTA) multicenter group.
IUD locations. See Intrauterine device (IUD) locations, abnormal.

K
Kidney, pelvic, 159–160
    clinical aspects of, 159
    differential diagnosis for, 159
    etiology of, 159
    recommendations for, 159
    synonyms of, 159
    ultrasound findings for, 159, 159f–160f
Kidney stones, 203. See also Ureteral stones.

L
Latzko triad, 196
Leiomyomas, 85
    benign metastasizing, 114. See also Intravenous leiomyomatosis.
    bladder, 15. See also Bladder masses.
    fibroids, 85–92. See also Fibroids.

Leiomyomatosis, intravenous, 114–115
    clinical aspects of, 115
    differential diagnosis for, 115
    etiology of, 114
    recommendations for, 115
    synonyms for, 114
    ultrasound findings for, 114
Leiomyosarcomas, 205. See also Uterine sarcomas.
Lesions
    anterior abdominal wall, 77–78. See also Endometriosis.
    bladder wall, 77–78
    focal bladder, 15
LMPs. See Low malignant potential tumors (LMPs).
Locations, intrauterine devices (IUDs), 109–113. See also Abnormal intrauterine device (IUD) locations.
Low malignant potential tumors (LMPs), 21. See also Borderline ovarian tumor.
Lymph nodes, enlarged, 116–117
    clinical aspects of, 116
    differential diagnosis for, 116
    etiology of, 116
    recommendations for, 116
    synonyms for, 116
    ultrasound findings for, 116, 116f–117f
Lymphomas, bowel, 27. See also Bowel diseases.

M
Malignant germ cell tumors, 56. See also Dysgerminomas.
Malignant mixed Müllerian tumors (MMMTs), 205–208. See also Uterine sarcomas.
Masses
    appendiceal, 11. See also Appendiceal mucocele.
    bladder, 15–20
    cervical, 34–38
    vaginal, 209–218
Massive edema, 147–152
    clinical aspects of, 148
    differential diagnosis for, 147
    etiology of, 147
    recommendations for, 148
    synonyms for, 147
    ultrasound findings for, 147, 148f–151f
Mature teratomas
    cystic, 53. See also Dermoid cysts.
    monophyletic, 83. See also Epidermoid cysts.
Menopause, early, 170. See also Premature ovarian failure (POF).
Mesothelial cysts, 155. See also Paratubal and paraovarian cysts.
Mesotheliomas, benign cystic, 8. See also Adhesions.
Metastasizing leiomyomas, benign, 114. See also Intravenous leiomyomatosis.
Metastatic tumors to ovaries, 118–121. See also Tumors.
    clinical aspects of, 118
    differential diagnosis for, 118
    etiology of, 118
    recommendations for, 118
    synonyms for, 118
    ultrasound findings for, 118, 119f–121f
Mirena intrauterine device (IUD), 109. See also Intrauterine device (IUD) locations, abnormal.
Mixed epithelial and mesenchymal tumors, 205. See also Uterine sarcomas.
MMMTs. See Malignant mixed Müllerian tumors (MMMTs).
Monodermal highly specialized mature cystic teratomas, 186. See also Struma ovarii.
Monophyletic teratomas, mature, 83. See also Epidermoid cysts.

Mucinous cystadenomas, 122–124. *See also* Cystadenomas.
  clinical aspects of, 122–123
  differential diagnosis for, 122
  etiology of, 122
  recommendations for, 122–123
  synonyms for, 122
  ultrasound findings for, 122, 123f
Mucocele, appendiceal, 11–13. *See also* Appendiceal mucocele.
Müllerian duct anomalies, 125–135
  classification of, 125
  etiology of, 125
  synonyms for, 125
  ultrasound findings for, 126, 127f–135f
Myomas, 85. *See also* Fibroids.
Myometrium
  endometriosis of, 3. *See also* Adenomyosis.
  intracavity scan protocols, 225–226

N

Nephrolithiasis, 203. *See also* Ureteral stones.
Nonfunctional cysts, 43. *See also* Corpus luteum (CL).
Nongynecologic organs, 232–233
Normal anatomy, 221–223
Normal pelvic scans and variants, 219–234
  anatomy, normal, 221–223
  intracavity scan protocols, 221–223
    adnexa, 221, 229–231, 232f
    cervix, 20f, 224, 225f
    cul-de-sac, 225f, 231–232
    endometrium, 224–229, 227f–228f
    myometrium, 225–226
    ovaries, 229–231, 232f–233f
    perineum, 18f, 223–224
    uterus, 221, 222f–223f, 224–229, 225f–226f
    vagina, 223–224, 224f
  nongynecologic organs, 232–233
  quality-related considerations of, 232–233
  techniques, 221–223
    probe disinfection, 221–222
    transabdominal (TA) scans, 221–223, 222f
    transrectal (TR) scans, 222, 223f
    transvaginal (TV) scans, 221–223, 223f

O

Organs, nongynecologic, 232–233
Ovarian calcifications, 136. *See also* Calcifications, ovarian.
Ovarian cancer
  borderline, 21–25
    clinical aspects of, 21
    differential diagnosis for, 21
    etiology of, 21
    recommendations for, 21
    synonyms for, 21
    ultrasound findings for, 21, 22f–25f
  epithelial, 137–146
    clinical aspects of, 138
    differential diagnosis for, 138
    etiology of, 137
    recommendations for, 138
    synonyms for, 137
    ultrasound findings for, 11, 137–138, 139f–145f
  International Ovarian Tumor Analysis (IOTA) multicenter group and, 138
  metastatic tumors, 118–121
Ovarian cysts, clear, 48. *See also* Clear cysts.
Ovarian failure, premature, 170–171. *See also* Premature ovarian failure (POF).
Ovarian fibromas, 93–95
  clinical aspects of, 93
  differential diagnosis for, 93
  etiology of, 93
  recommendations for, 93
  synonyms for, 93
  ultrasound findings for, 93, 93f–95f

Ovarian insufficiency, 170. *See also* Premature ovarian failure (POF).
Ovarian metastatic tumors, 118–121. *See also* Metastatic tumors to ovaries.
Ovarian pregnancies, 58. *See also* Ectopic pregnancies.
Ovarian sebaceous cysts, 83. *See also* Epidermoid cysts.
Ovarian torsion, 147–152
  clinical aspects of, 148
  differential diagnosis for, 147
  etiology of, 147
  recommendations for, 148
  synonyms for, 147
  ultrasound findings for, 147, 148f–151f
Ovarian vein thrombosis, 153–154
  clinical aspects of, 153
  differential diagnosis for, 153
  etiology of, 153
  recommendations for, 153
  synonyms of, 153
  ultrasound findings for, 56, 153, 154f
Ovaries, polycystic, 161–162. *See also* Polycystic ovarian syndrome (PCOS).

P

ParaGard intrauterine device (IUD), 109. *See also* Intrauterine device (IUD) locations, abnormal.
Paramesonephric cysts, 155. *See also* Paratubal and paraovarian cysts.
Paraovarian cysts. *See* Paratubal and paraovarian cysts
Paratubal and paraovarian cysts, 155–156. *See also* Cysts.
  clinical aspects of, 155
  differential diagnosis for, 155
  etiology of, 155
  recommendations for, 155
  synonyms for, 155
  ultrasound findings for, 155, 155f–156f
PCOS. *See* Polycystic ovarian syndrome (PCOS)
Pedunculated fibroids, 85. *See also* Fibroids.
Pelvic abscesses, 199. *See also* Pelvic inflammatory disease (PID).
Pelvic congestion syndrome, 157–158
  clinical aspects of, 157
  differential diagnosis for, 157
  etiology of, 157
  recommendations for, 157
  synonyms for, 157
  ultrasound findings for, 157, 157f
Pelvic infections, 199. *See also* Pelvic inflammatory disease (PID).
Pelvic inflammatory disease (PID), 199–202
  clinical aspects of, 199–200
  differential diagnosis for, 199
  etiology of, 199
  recommendations for, 199–200
  synonyms for, 199
  vs. tubo-ovarian abscesses (TOAs), 199
  ultrasound findings for, 199, 200f–202f
Pelvic kidney, 159–160
  clinical aspects of, 159
  differential diagnosis for, 159
  etiology of, 159
  recommendations for, 159
  synonyms of, 159
  ultrasound findings for, 159, 159f–160f
Pelvic varicose veins, 157. *See also* Pelvic congestion syndrome.
Peritoneal inclusion cysts, 8–10
  clinical aspects of, 8
  differential diagnosis for, 8
  etiology of, 8
  recommendations for, 8
  synonyms for, 8
  ultrasound findings for, 8, 9f–10f

PFTCs. *See* Primary fallopian tube carcinomas (PFTCs)
PID. *See* Pelvic inflammatory disease (PID)
Placenta, retained, 172. *See also* Retained products of conception (RPOC).
POF. *See* Premature ovarian failure (POF)
Polycystic ovarian syndrome (PCOS), 161–162
  clinical aspects of, 161
  differential diagnosis for, 161
  etiology of, 161
  recommendations for, 161
  synonyms for, 161
  ultrasound findings for, 161, 162f
Polyps
  endometrial, 163–169
    clinical aspects of, 163
    differential diagnosis for, 163
    etiology of, 163
    recommendations for, 163
    synonyms for, 163
    ultrasound findings for, 163, 164f–169f
  hyperplastic, 163
  proliferative, 163
Postmenopausal clear cysts, 48. *See also* Clear cysts.
Pregnancies, ectopic, 58–64
  clinical aspects of, 59
  differential diagnosis for, 59
  etiology of, 58
  recommendations for, 59
  synonyms for, 58
  ultrasound findings for, 58–59, 60f–64f
Pregnancy of unknown location (PUL), 58. *See also* Ectopic pregnancies.
Premature ovarian failure (POF), 170–171
  clinical aspects of, 170
  differential diagnosis for, 170
  etiology of, 170
  recommendations for, 170
  synonyms for, 170
  ultrasound findings for, 170, 171f
Premenopausal clear cysts, 48. *See also* Clear cysts.
Primary fallopian tube carcinomas (PFTCs), 196–198. *See also* Carcinomas.
  BRCA 1/BRCA 2 and, 196
  clinical aspects of, 196
  differential diagnosis for, 196
  etiology of, 196
  Latzko triad and, 196
  recommendations for, 196
  serous intraepithelial tubal carcinomas (STICs) and, 196
  synonyms for, 196
  ultrasound findings for, 196, 197f–198f
Probe disinfection, 221–222
Proliferation, endometrial, 71. *See also* Endometrial hyperplasia.
Proliferative polyps, 163
PUL. *See* Pregnancy of unknown location (PUL).
Pyocolpos, 98. *See also* Hematometra and hematocolpos.
Pyometra, 98. *See also* Hematometra and hematocolpos.

Q
Quality-related considerations, 232–233

R
Rectosigmoid colon, endometriosis of, 26. *See also* Bowel diseases.
Renal stones, 203. *See also* Ureteral stones.
Retained placenta, 172. *See also* Retained products of conception (RPOC).
Retained products of conception (RPOC), 172–176
  Asherman's syndrome and, 177–178. *See also* Asherman's syndrome.

Retained products of conception (Continued)
  clinical aspects of, 172–173
  differential diagnosis for, 172
  etiology of, 172
  recommendations for, 172–173
  synonyms of, 172
  ultrasound findings for, 172, 173f–176f
RPOC. See Retained products of conception
  (RPOC)

S
SAB. See Spontaneous abortion (SAB), incomplete.
Sarcomas, uterine, 205–208
  classification of, 205
  clinical aspects of, 206
  differential diagnosis for, 205
  etiology of, 205
  recommendations for, 206
  synonyms for, 205
  ultrasound findings for, 205, 207f–208f
Scar defects, Cesarean section (C-section), 39–42.
  See also Cesarean section (C-section) scar
  defects.
Schwann cell tumors. See Schwannomas.
Schwannomas, 182–183
  clinical aspects of, 182
  differential diagnosis for, 182
  etiology of, 182
  recommendations for, 182
  synonyms of, 182
  ultrasound findings for, 182, 183f
Sebaceous cysts of ovary, 83. See also Epidermoid
  cysts.
Septate uterus, 125. See also Müllerian duct
  anomalies.
Septic pelvic thrombophlebitis (SPT), 153. See also
  Ovarian vein thrombosis.
Serous cystadenomas, 184–185. See also
  Cystadenomas.
  clinical aspects of, 184
  differential diagnosis for, 184
  etiology of, 184
  recommendations for, 184
  synonyms for, 184
  ultrasound findings for, 184, 184f–185f
Serous intraepithelial tubal carcinomas (STICs),
  137. See also Epithelial ovarian cancer.
Sex-cord-gonadal stromal tumors, 96. See also
  Granulosa cell tumors (GCTs).
Simple cysts, 48. See also Clear cysts.
Solid masses, vaginal, 209. See also Vaginal cysts.
Spontaneous abortion (SAB), incomplete, 172. See
  also Retained products of conception (RPOC).
SPT. See Septic pelvic thrombophlebitis (SPT).
STICs. See Serous intraepithelial tubal carcinomas
  (STICs)
Stones, ureteral, 203–204
  clinical aspects of, 203
  differential diagnosis for, 203
  etiology of, 203
  recommendations for, 203
  synonyms for, 203
  ultrasound findings for, 203, 204f
Stromal tumors
  cystadenomas
    mucinous, 122–124
    serous, 184–185
  fibromas, ovarian, 93–95
  fibrothecomas, 93–95
  gastrointestinal (GISTs), 27
  thecomas, 93–95
  World Health Organization (WHO) classifica-
    tion of, 93
Struma ovarii, 186–188
  clinical aspects of, 186
  differential diagnosis for, 186
  etiology of, 186

Struma ovarii (Continued)
  recommendations for, 186
  synonyms for, 186
  ultrasound findings for, 186, 187f–188f
Submucous fibroids, 85. See also Fibroids.
Subserosal fibroids, 85. See also Fibroids.
Syndromes
  Asherman's, 177–181
  pelvic congestion, 157–158
  polycystic ovarian syndrome (PCOS), 161
Synechiae, 177. See also Asherman's syndrome.

T
TA scans. See Transabdominal (TA) scans.
TAB. See Therapeutic abortion (TAB).
Tarlov cysts, 192–193. See also Cysts.
  clinical aspects of, 192
  differential diagnosis for, 192
  etiology of, 192
  recommendations for, 192
  synonyms for, 192
  ultrasound findings for, 192, 192f–193f
Techniques, 221–223
  probe disinfection, 221–222
  transabdominal (TA) scans, 221–223, 222f
  transrectal (TR) scans, 222, 223f
  transvaginal (TV) scans, 221–223, 223f
Teratomas
  cystic, 53. See also Dermoid cysts.
  mature
    monodermal highly specialized cystic, 186.
      See also Struma ovarii.
    monophyletic, 83. See also Epidermoid cysts.
Theca lutein cysts, 194–195. See also Cysts.
  clinical aspects of, 194
  differential diagnosis for, 194
  etiology of, 194
  human chorionic gonadotropin (hCG) and, 194
  recommendations for, 194
  synonyms for, 194
  ultrasound findings for, 194, 194f–195f
Thecomas, 93–95
  clinical aspects of, 93
  differential diagnosis for, 93
  etiology of, 93
  fibrothecomas, 93–95. See also Fibrothecomas.
  recommendations for, 93
  synonyms for, 93
  ultrasound findings for, 93, 93f–95f
Therapeutic abortion (TAB), 177
Thick endometrium, differential diagnosis, 71–75
Thrombosis, ovarian vein, 153–154
  clinical aspects of, 153
  differential diagnosis for, 153
  etiology of, 153
  recommendations for, 153
  synonyms of, 153
  ultrasound findings for, 56, 153, 154f
TOAs. See Tubo-ovarian abscesses (TOAs)
Torsion, ovarian/tubal, 147–152
  clinical aspects of, 148
  differential diagnosis for, 147
  etiology of, 147
  recommendations for, 148
  synonyms for, 147
  ultrasound findings for, 147, 148f–151f
TR scans. See Transrectal (TR) scans.
Transabdominal (TA) scans, 221–223, 222f
Transitional cell tumors
  of bladder, 15. See also Bladder masses.
  of ovaries, 32. See also Brenner tumors.
Transrectal (TR) scans, 222, 223f
Transvaginal (TV) scans, 221–223, 223f
T-shaped uterus, 189–191
  Asherman's syndrome and, 189. See also Asher-
    man's syndrome.
  clinical aspects of, 189

T-shaped uterus (Continued)
  diethylstilbestrol (DES) and, 189
  differential diagnosis for, 189
  etiology of, 189
  recommendations for, 189
  synonyms for, 189
  ultrasound findings for, 189, 190f–191f
Tubal carcinomas, 196. See also Primary fallopian
  tube carcinomas (PFTCs).
Tubal pregnancies, 58. See also Ectopic
  pregnancies.
Tubal torsion, 147–152
  clinical aspects of, 148
  differential diagnosis for, 147
  etiology of, 147
  recommendations for, 148
  synonyms for, 147
  ultrasound findings for, 147, 148f–151f
Tubo-ovarian abscesses (TOAs), 199–202
  clinical aspects of, 199–200
  differential diagnosis for, 199
  etiology of, 199
  vs. pelvic inflammatory disease (PID), 199–200
  recommendations for, 199–200
  synonyms for, 199
  ultrasound findings for, 199, 200f–202f
Tumors
  bladder, 15
  Brenner, 32–33
  gastrointestinal stromal (GISTs), 27
  germ cell, benign vs. malignant, 56
  granulosa cell (GCTs), 96–97
  low malignant potential (LMPs), 21
  metastatic to ovaries, 118–121
  stromal. See Stromal tumors
  transitional cell. See Transitional cell tumors.
TV scans. See Transvaginal (TV) scans.

U
Ulcerative colitis, 26. See also Bowel diseases.
Ultrasound, gynecologic
  of entities
    abscesses, tubo-ovarian (TOAs), 199–202
    adenomyosis, 1–7
    adhesions, 8–10
    bowel diseases, 26–31
    calcifications, ovarian, 136
    carcinomas, endometrial, 65–70
    carcinomas, primary fallopian tube (PFTCs),
      196–198
    Cesarean section (C-section) scar defects,
      39–42
    corpus luteum (CL), 43–47
    cystadenofibromas, 51–52
    cystadenomas, mucinous, 122–124
    cystadenomas, serous, 184–185
    cysts, clear, 48–50
    cysts, dermoid, 53–55
    cysts, paraovarian, 155–156
    cysts, paratubal, 155–156
    cysts, peritoneal inclusion, 8–10
    cysts, Tarlov, 192–193
    cysts, theca lutein, 194–195
    dehiscence, uterine, 39–42
    dysgerminomas, 56–57
    edema, massive, 147–152
    endometriosis, 76–82
    endometrium, atrophic, 14
    endometrium, thick (differential diagnosis),
      71–75
    fibroids, 85–92
    fibromas, ovarian, 93–95
    fibrothecomas, 93–95
    hematocolpos, 98–103
    hematometra, 98–103
    hematuria, 15–20
    hydrosalpinx, 104–108

Ultrasound, gynecologic (*Continued*)
 hyperplasia, endometrial, 71–75
 intrauterine device (IUD) locations, abnormal, 109–113
 leiomyomatosis, intravenous, 114–115
 lymph nodes, enlarged, 116–117
 masses, bladder, 15–20
 masses, cervical, 34–38
 masses, vaginal, 209–218
 mucocele, appendiceal, 11–13
 Müllerian duct abnormalities, 125–135
 ovarian cancer, epithelial, 137–146
 ovarian tumor, borderline, 21–25
 pelvic inflammatory disease (PID), 199–202
 pelvic kidney, 159–160
 polycystic ovaries, 161–162
 polyps, endometrial, 163–169
 pregnancies, ectopic, 58–64
 premature ovarian failure, 170–171
 retained products of conception (RPOC), 172–176
 sarcomas, uterine, 205–208
 Schwannomas, 182–183
 stones, ureteral, 203–204
 struma ovarii, 186–188
 syndrome, Asherman's, 177–181
 syndrome, pelvic congestion, 157–158
 thecomas, 93–95
 torsion, ovarian, 147–152
 torsion, tubal, 147–152
 tumors, Brenner, 32–33
 tumors, granulosa cell (GCTs), 96–97
 tumors, metastatic to ovaries, 118–121
 uterus, T-shaped, 189–191
 vein thrombosis, ovarian, 153–154

Ultrasound, gynecologic (*Continued*)
 normal pelvic scans and variants, 219–234
 anatomy, normal, 221–223
 intracavity scan protocols, 223–232. *See also*
 Intracavity scan protocols.
 nongynecologic organs, 232–233
 quality-related considerations of, 232–233
 techniques, 221–223. *See also* Techniques.
Unicornuate uterus, 125. *See also* Müllerian duct
 anomalies.
Ureteral stones, 203–204
 clinical aspects of, 203
 differential diagnosis for, 203
 etiology of, 203
 recommendations for, 203
 synonyms for, 203
 ultrasound findings for, 203, 204f
Urethral diverticula, 15. *See also* Bladder masses.
Uterine cancer, 65. *See also* Endometrial carcinomas.
Uterine dehiscence, 39–42
 clinical aspects of, 39
 differential diagnosis for, 39
 etiology of, 39
 recommendations for, 39
 synonyms for, 39
 ultrasound findings for, 39, 40f–41f
Uterine fibromas, 85. *See also* Fibroids.
Uterine sarcomas, 205–208
 classification of, 205
 clinical aspects of, 206
 differential diagnosis for, 205
 etiology of, 205
 recommendations for, 206
 synonyms for, 205
 ultrasound findings for, 205, 207f–208f

Uterus
 anatomy, normal, 221–223
 endometriosis of, 3. *See also* Adenomyosis.
 intracavity scan protocols, 221, 222f–223f, 224–229, 225f–226f

V
Vagina
 anatomy, normal, 221–223
 intracavity scan protocols, 223–224, 224f
Vaginal cysts, 209. *See also* Vaginal masses.
Vaginal masses, 209–218. *See also* Masses.
 clinical aspects of, 210
 cysts, 209
 differential diagnosis for, 210
 etiology of, 209
 recommendations for, 210
 solid masses, 209
 synonyms for, 209
 ultrasound findings for, 209, 211f–217f
Varicose veins, pelvic, 157. *See also* Pelvic congestion syndrome.
Vein thrombosis, ovarian, 153–154
 clinical aspects of, 153
 differential diagnosis for, 153
 etiology of, 153
 recommendations for, 153
 synonyms of, 153
 ultrasound findings for, 56, 153, 154f

W
World Health Organization (WHO) classifications, 93